Urology

AN ILLUSTRATED COLOUR TEXT

Commissioning Editor: Timothy Horne
Project Development Manager: Lulu Stader
Project Manager: Jess Thompson
Design Direction: Erik Bigland
Illustration Manager: Bruce Hogarth
Illustrator: Amanda Williams

Urology

AN ILLUSTRATED COLOUR TEXT

Nigel Bullock MD FRCS
Consultant Urologist, Addenbrooke's NHS Trust, Cambridge, UK
Associate Lecturer, University of Cambridge, UK

Andrew Doble MB BS MS FRCS (Urol)
Consultant Urologist, Addenbrooke's NHS Trust, Cambridge, UK
Associate Lecturer, University of Cambridge, UK

William Turner MA MD FRCS (Urol)
Consultant Urologist, Addenbrooke's NHS Trust, Cambridge, UK
Associate Lecturer, University of Cambridge, UK

Peter Cuckow MB BS FRCS (Paed)
Consultant Paediatric Urologist, Great Ormond Street and Middlesex
Hospital, London, UK

Illustrated by Amanda Williams

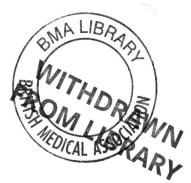
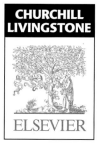
CHURCHILL
LIVINGSTONE

ELSEVIER

EDINBURGH   LONDON   NEW YORK   OXFORD   PHILADELPHIA   ST LOUIS   SYDNEY   TORONTO   2008

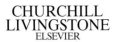

CHURCHILL
LIVINGSTONE
ELSEVIER

© Elsevier Limited 2008

The right of Nigel Bullock, Andrew Doble, William Turner and
Peter Cuckow to be identified as authors of this work has been asserted
by them in accordance with the Copyright, Designs and Patents Act 1988.

First Edition 2008
  Reprinted 2008

ISBN 978-0-443-07264-2

British Library Cataloguing in Publication Data
A catalogue record for this book is available from the British Library

Library of Congress Cataloging in Publication Data
A catalog record for this book is available from the Library of Congress

ELSEVIER your source for books,
journals and multimedia
in the health sciences
www.elsevierhealth.com

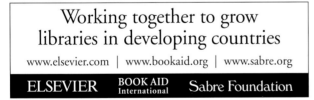

Working together to grow
libraries in developing countries

www.elsevier.com | www.bookaid.org | www.sabre.org

ELSEVIER BOOK AID International Sabre Foundation

The
publisher's
policy is to use
**paper manufactured
from sustainable forests**

Printed in China

Preface

Urology is a young specialty with a short history. It arrived as a specialty in its own right with the development of the rigid Hopkins® lens system in the 1950s; this allowed urologists to perform procedures endoscopically that, hitherto, had been carried out as open operations, often with significant morbidity and mortality. Since then, there has been a proliferation of new techniques, mostly in the area of minimally invasive surgery, so that we can now examine every area of the urinary tract endoscopically and perform procedures without incisions in the majority of our patients. It has been a constant challenge, even for the specialist urologist, to keep up with the rapid progress in these new techniques.

At the same time, a better understanding of the natural history of urological diseases such as prostate cancer, bladder cancer and infertility has resulted in major changes in the way urological disease is now managed. Research in molecular biology has improved our understanding of disease processes, especially malignancy, and will eventually allow us to implement treatments for urological cancers on a more logical basis.

This book aims to summarise all these recent advances by describing current practice in urological surgery in a simple, concise and comprehensible manner. The rapid development of new treatment modalities means that new techniques will continue to be introduced, rendering every textbook out of date by the time it has been written. This is particularly so in a progressive specialty such as urology, so we have attempted to provide an insight not only into the present but also into what the future holds. For urological surgeons, the future has never been so exciting.

Adrian Wagg cowrote the pages on incontinence in the elderly. Without the help, advice and contributions of our professional colleagues, both physicians and surgeons, this book would never have been possible, and we gratefully acknowledge the contributions they have all made.

KNB, PC, AD, WHT

Contents

Tumours of the Genitourinary Tract 107

Benign Genital Disorders 135

Structure and Function of the Genitourinary Tract

Embryology and development of the urinary tract

Introduction

During the first 10 weeks of gestation (embryonic phase), the genitourinary organs develop from primitive precursor cells in the intermediate mesoderm of the embryonic disc. They then grow and develop function over the next 28 weeks (fetal phase).

Development of the bladder and kidneys

By the fifth week of gestation, the embryonic disc has folded, and the precursors of the urogenital system are clearly visible. Above the tail fold, a midline cavity (cloaca) forms from the urogenital sinus anteriorly and the hindgut posteriorly. On either side, the mesonephros and the gonads develop, while the mesonephric and paramesonephric ducts run down to the back of the urogenital sinus. At their lower ends, the paramesonephric (Müllerian) ducts fuse at the Müllerian tubercle; this will eventually form the female uterus. Above this, ureteric buds develop and grow outwards from the mesonephric ducts to fuse with a group of blastema cells, which form the metanephros (kidney). The septum divides the cloaca to separate the urogenital sinus anteriorly and the developing rectum posteriorly.

By the sixth week of gestation, the kidneys are forming with the ureteric buds dividing to form the distal nephrons and the blastema cells differentiating to form glomeruli. The distal mesonephric ducts are absorbed into the urogenital sinus so that the origins of the ureteric buds also drain directly into the sinus. The genital tubercle is starting to develop anteriorly, and the cloacal membrane faces in a more downwards direction.

By the eighth week of gestation, the urorectal septum is complete. The kidney ascends from the pelvis and rotates internally so the renal pelvis faces anteromedially. The lower ends of the mesonephric duct and ureter are further incorporated into the posterior wall of the urogenital sinus. Their orientation changes so they enter the developing bladder above and lateral to the mesonephric ducts; the triangular area between them becomes the trigone.

Development of the internal genitalia

The gonads form from primitive germ cells interacting with the intermediate mesoderm, and these lie anterior to the mesonephros (Fig. 1). There is little discernible difference between male and female until the sixth week of gestation.

In females, the ovaries arise from the cortex of the indifferent gonad, and the fallopian tubes/body of the uterus from the paramesonephric (Müllerian) ducts. The mesonephric (Wolffian) ducts degenerate leaving vestigial remnants. The ovaries descend into the pelvis, and remnants of the gubernacula form the round ligaments. The upper vagina forms from the paramesonephric ducts and the lower vagina from the urogenital sinus.

In males, the presence of testis-determining factor forces the indifferent gonad to differentiate into the body of the testis and the mesonephric duct into its collecting system (the epididymis, vas and seminal vesicles). The testis produces Müllerian-inhibiting substance so that the Müllerian duct system regresses, leaving a vestigial appendage to the epididymis and a small utricule in the prostatic urethra. Testosterone stimulates differentiation of the duct system from the mesonephric duct. The gubernacula remain the same length and draw the testes downwards as the fetus grows.

At around 6 months, an extension of the abdominal cavity (the processus vaginalis) passes through the muscle wall of the abdomen towards the developing scrotal sacs. The testis

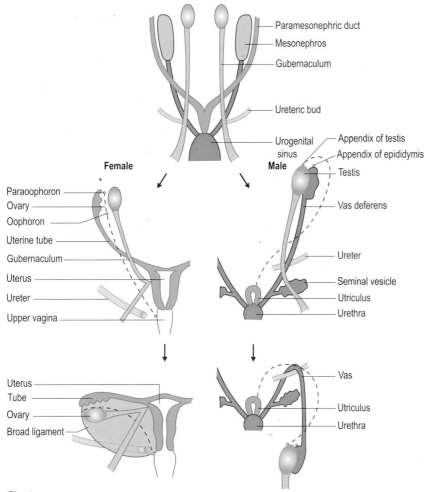

Fig. 1 **Development of the internal genitalia.**

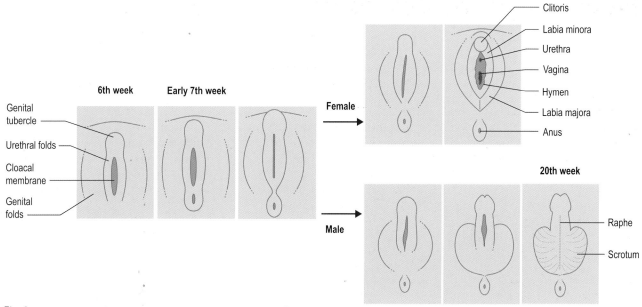

Fig. 2 **Development of the external genitalia.**

descends inside the processus vaginalis, which then loses its attachment to the abdominal cavity. This process is complete by the end of the eighth month of gestation.

Development of the external genitalia

Development of the external genitalia begins from the indifferent phase between the sixth and seventh weeks of gestation (Fig. 2).

Development of urinary tract function

By the midpoint of gestation, the kidneys are producing urine, the bladder is already filling and emptying (cycling) about once an hour, and bladder volume increases as gestation progresses. After birth, voiding is by spinal reflex about once an hour, gradually decreasing over the first year to about 10 times

daily. After 1 year, the child learns to inhibit this reflex, and voluntary control is gradually imposed. Adult-pattern micturition is usually achieved after 3 or 4 years due to lower urinary

tract development and adaptation of reflex voiding by higher cognitive function. Bladder capacity then increases progressively throughout childhood.

Table 1 Embryological origins of anomalies of the urinary tract

Organ system	Problem	Result
Kidneys	Failure of fusion of ureteric bud with blastema	Dysplastic or poorly functioning kidney
	Failure of ascent	Ectopic or pelvic kidney
	Fusion of the developing kidneys	Horseshoe kidney or fused kidneys
Ureters	Failure of ureteric bud	Renal agenesis and hemitrigone
	Two ureteric buds	Duplex kidney and collecting system
	Abnormal ureteric bud origin	Ectopic or abnormally placed ureteric orifice
Bladder	Rupture of cloacal membrane	Bladder exstrophy
	Failure of septation of cloaca	Cloacal anomaly
	Rupture of cloacal membrane and failure of septation	Cloacal exstrophy
Female internal genitalia	Failure of Müllerian midline fusion	Bifid vagina or uterus
Male internal genitalia	Failure of testicular descent	Undescended or impalpable testis
Female external genitalia	Inappropriate testosterone production	Ambiguous genitalia (congenital adrenal hyperplasia)
Male external genitalia	Incomplete fusion	Hypospadias
	Absent/no response to testosterone	Female appearance or severe hypospadias

---

Key points

- Embryological development of the genitourinary tract is a complex series of events occurring primarily within the first 8 weeks of gestation.
- The internal and external genitalia develop from indifferent structures under sex-related inhibitory and stimulatory factors.
- Congenital abnormalities of the genitourinary tract can be explained by a detailed understanding of embryological development (Table 1).
- Development of the lower urinary tract in particular continues after birth.

Anatomy of the urinary tract

Kidneys

Macroscopic structure

The kidneys lie on the posterior abdominal wall, the right kidney lying slightly lower than the left; they are covered anteriorly by abdominal organs (Fig. 1). The medial border of the kidney forms the hilum with the renal vein anteriorly, the artery behind it and the renal pelvis lying posteriorly. The renal pelvis divides into three or four major calyces, which in turn divide into a number of minor calyces, each indented by a medullary pyramid. The kidneys are surrounded by Gerota's fascia, which is incomplete inferiorly. Arterial supply is directly from the aorta by a single renal artery, but accessory arteries are common; the intrarenal arteries are strictly segmental. Venous drainage is directly into the inferior vena cava (IVC) but is not segmental. Nerve supply is from T12 and L1 (sympathetic) and from the vagus nerve.

Microscopic structure

The functional unit of the kidney is the nephron (Fig. 2). The *glomerulus* lies within the renal cortex in a glomerular (*Bowman's*) capsule and is supplied with blood by a tuft of capillaries through which filtration occurs; branches of the efferent arterioles also supply the renal medulla (*vasa recta*). The filtrate passes through the nephron, undergoing substantial modification as it progresses, and is released through the collecting tubules into larger collecting ducts (*ducts of Bellini*). Where the distal tubule of each nephron lies close to its glomerulus, its walls are thickened to form a *macula densa*, and the afferent arteriolar walls are hypertrophied to form the *juxtaglomerular apparatus*.

Surgery and the kidney

The kidneys are best approached via a loin incision through the bed of the 11th or 12th rib, but large renal tumours are generally approached via a transperitoneal approach, although much renal surgery is now accomplished by laparoscopy. Because Gerota's fascia is incomplete below the kidney, urine or blood from the kidney can track down around the upper ureter. Removal of the right kidney tends to be more difficult because the right renal vein is often very short and prone to tear during surgery.

Ureters

Macroscopic structure

The ureter is a muscular tube designed for peristalsis. It is adherent to the back of the peritoneum and passes down to the level of the ischial spine, where it turns medially to enter the bladder (Fig. 3), passing above the seminal vesicle in men and below the uterine artery and broad ligament in women. Entry into the bladder is oblique for the last 2 cm to prevent vesicoureteric reflux. Blood supply is largely segmental, but becomes more tenuous in the lower ureter. Innervation is from the renal, aortic and hypogastric plexuses.

Microscopic structure

The ureter consists of an outer adventitial layer, smooth muscle and a lining of transitional epithelium supported by a *lamina propria*. In the upper ureter, the outer muscle is circular, whereas the inner fibres are oblique; longitudinal fibres predominate further down the ureter and are most apparent at the ureterovesical junction. Although there are no ganglion cells in the ureteric wall, there is a rich autonomic nerve supply.

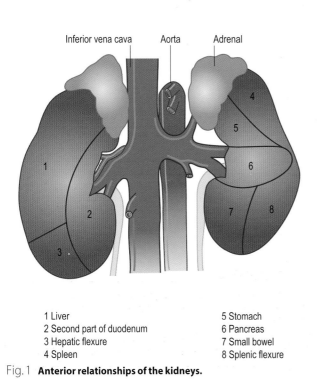

1 Liver
2 Second part of duodenum
3 Hepatic flexure
4 Spleen
5 Stomach
6 Pancreas
7 Small bowel
8 Splenic flexure

Fig. 1 **Anterior relationships of the kidneys.**

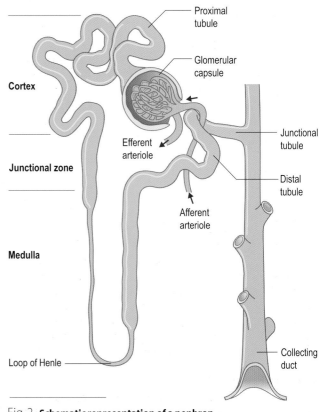

Fig. 2 **Schematic representation of a nephron.**

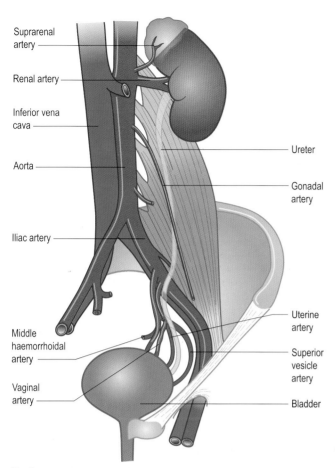

Suprarenal artery

Renal artery

Inferior vena cava

Aorta

Iliac artery

Middle haemorrhoidal artery

Vaginal artery

Ureter

Gonadal artery

Uterine artery

Superior vesicle artery

Bladder

Fig. 3 **Retroperitoneal course of the ureter.**

Surgery and the ureter

Urologists usually approach the lumen of the ureter retrogradely by flexible or rigid ureteroscopy. If open surgery is required, the upper third of the ureter is exposed in the same way as the kidney, the middle third of the ureter via a retroperitoneal, muscle-splitting incision and the lower third by a Pfannenstiel or midline incision with division of the superior vesical pedicle to facilitate exposure. The ureter can be identified during abdominal surgery by peristaltic movement on direct stimulation (*vermiculation*). The narrowest part of the ureter is the ureterovesical junction, and this is where calculi most often impact. The female ureter is most often damaged during division of the ureterine artery where it lies below the broad ligament; it is also at this site that a ureteric calculus may be felt on vaginal examination.

Bladder

Macroscopic structure

The bladder lies anteriorly in the pelvis bounded by the pubic bone and the pelvic side-walls. Its upper aspect is covered by peritoneum, leaving a retropubic space (*cave of Retzius*) anteriorly. Blood supply is from the anterior branch of the internal iliac artery via superior and inferior vesical arteries. Innervation is from pelvic parasympathetics (S2–S4) and from the hypogastric plexus (sympathetic).

Microscopic structure

The bladder is composed of a network of smooth muscle (*detrusor muscle*) lined by transitional epithelium. At the base of the bladder lies the *trigone*, bounded by the internal urethral orifice and the two ureteric openings. In men, the bladder neck forms a distinct sphincter but, in women, there is no corresponding sphincter.

Surgery and the bladder

Surgical procedures on the bladder are usually performed via the urethra using endoscopes. The extraperitoneal position of the bladder allows it to rise out of the pelvis and permits open surgery or percutaneous catheterisation via a lower abdominal incision without crossing the peritoneal cavity. Trauma to the bladder is usually extraperitoneal, but rupture can occur into the abdominal cavity.

Urethra

Macroscopic structure

The male urethra is divided into prostatic, membranous, bulbar and spongiose parts with the *navicular fossa* at the tip of the penis; the spongiose urethra is surrounded by the corpus spongiosum. The prostatic utricle and ejaculatory ducts open into the floor of the prostatic urethra, and the membranous urethra is the site of distal sphincter activity; the sphincter maintains normal continence and is part smooth muscle, part striated muscle (*rhabdosphincter*).

Microscopic structure

The urethra is lined by transitional epithelium as far as the navicular fossa, which has a squamous epithelium. Numerous mucin-secreting glands open into the female urethra and the male spongiose part.

Surgery and the urethra

The urethra is usually approached endoscopically, but open surgery is by direct incision through the perineum in men, dividing the bulbar muscles, or through the anterior vaginal wall in women. The male urethra can be injured in the perineum by direct trauma, resulting in a typical 'butterfly' haematoma.

> *Key points*
>
> ■ The anatomical relationships of the main organs of the urinary tract determine not only how they are approached surgically but also the effects that external trauma may have.
>
> ■ The kidneys, ureters and bladder may all be approached laparoscopically, by open surgery or endoscopically via their lumina.

Physiology of the urinary tract

The kidney

There are 1.5 million nephrons in each kidney, the majority lying superficially in the cortex of the kidney; a small proportion (*juxtamedullary nephrons*) lie deeper within the kidney and are important in the maintenance of ion concentrations. The basic functions of the kidney are shown in Table 1.

Filtering and volume regulation

Twenty-five per cent of the cardiac output (1200 mL/min) passes through the kidneys with 180 L of plasma being filtered each day; 99% of this is reabsorbed with only 1.5–1.8 L of urine being produced daily. Filtration is maintained over a range of arterial pressures between 75 mmHg and 160 mmHg by changes in the renal

Table 1 **Basic functions of the kidney**

Filtering and volume regulation
Maintenance of ion concentrations
Acid–base balance
Excretion of waste products
Endocrine functions

arterial resistance. These vascular changes may be influenced by local chemical release (e.g. prostaglandins, nitric oxide) but are primarily controlled by the sodium concentration in the macula densa; low levels trigger vasodilatation via the *juxtaglomerular apparatus* with activation of the *renin–angiotensin system*, vasoconstriction, aldosterone synthesis and, ultimately, sodium reabsorption. Water reabsorption is influenced by the action of antidiuretic hormone (ADH) on the distal tubules; ADH release by the posterior pituitary is triggered by osmoreceptors near the supraoptic nucleus that monitor plasma concentrations of sodium and chloride.

Maintenance of ion concentrations

Eighty per cent of filtered sodium and 90% of bicarbonate are reabsorbed in the proximal tubules. The tubular fluid remains isosmotic by simultaneous reabsorption of water and urea; potassium and sulphates are also reabsorbed in the proximal tubules. Sodium is reabsorbed from all parts of the loop of Henle, but water is only reabsorbed from the descending limb; this results in a concentration gradient in the renal medulla, which forms the basis of the *countercurrent multiplier system* to maintain water balance (Fig. 1). Seventy-five per cent of potassium excretion occurs by secretion from the distal tubules

Acid–base balance

Acid–base balance is controlled by complex buffer systems in the proximal and distal tubules, involving predominantly phosphate but also bicarbonate and ammonium ion buffering. Hydrogen ion secretion occurs predominantly in the distal tubule and occurs against a concentration gradient.

Excretion of waste products

The glomerular membrane allows molecules larger than 4 nm in diameter to pass through (equivalent to a molecular weight of 70 000). This allows waste products (e.g. urea, creatinine and urate) to be filtered, but does not permit the passage of proteins or blood cells. Glucose becomes a waste product only when its concentration in the plasma exceeds the capacity of the proximal tubule to reabsorb all the filtered glucose.

Endocrine functions

Erythropoietin is produced by the kidney in response to hypoxia, vasoconstriction and red cell breakdown. It stimulates the production of nucleated red cells in haemopoietic tissue. *Prostaglandins* are synthesised in the kidney, but their exact role in normal renal function is unclear. Vasodilator and vasoconstrictor prostaglandins are produced by a variety of stimuli, including raised pressure in Bowman's capsule. *Renin* is released from juxtaglomerular cells in response to poor tissue perfusion and converts angiotensinogen (from the liver) to angiotensin I; this is then converted by an enzyme (angiotensin-converting enzyme, ACE) to angiotensin II, which causes vasoconstriction, sodium reabsorption and restoration of tissue perfusion. *1,25-Dihydroxy-cholecalciferol*, the active metabolite of vitamin D, is produced in the kidneys and helps to maintain calcium levels. The kidneys also produce kinins such as *kallikrein* and *bradykinin*, which usually cause vasodilatation and result in increased urine flow with sodium excretion.

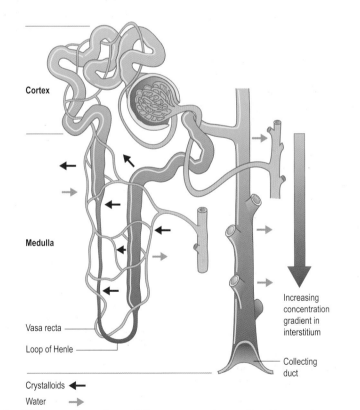

Cortex

Medulla

Vasa recta
Loop of Henle

Increasing concentration gradient in interstitium

Collecting duct

Crystalloids ◀
Water ▶

Fig. 1 **Establishment of a corticomedullary concentration gradient** (the countercurrent multiplier system).

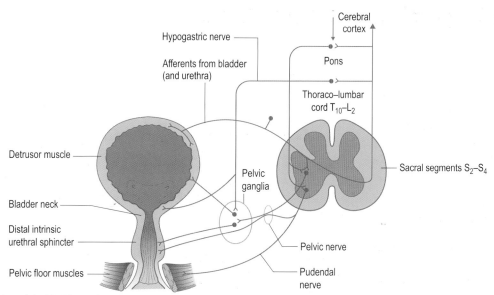

Fig. 2 **Innervation of the bladder and urethra.**

The ureter

The prime function of the ureter is *peristalsis*. Peristalsis is initiated in the minor calyces by morphologically distinct muscle cells that act as pacemakers. Each pacemaker fires in turn but does not always initiate a contraction wave. With higher urine flow, more pacemaker firings initiate contractions until, at high urine flow, all firings are effective. Myogenic contraction of the renal pelvis and ureter then results in bolus formation.

The first bolus is formed within the renal pelvis itself by a strong circular muscle contraction and by relaxation of the pelviureteric junction. Longitudinal contraction then lifts the ureter over the formed bolus, which moves downwards. Peristalsis is dependent on the capacity of the ureter to coapt its walls; obstruction, infection, atonic dilatation and ureteric instrumentation all inhibit coaption. Coaption of the ureter above a bolus prevents back-pressure being transmitted to the collecting system as urine passes down the ureter. At the bladder, longitudinal muscle contraction opens the ureteric orifice and allows urine to enter the bladder. The intramural ureter, together with ureteric coaption and the 'flutter valve' effect of urine in the bladder, prevents reflux of urine back up the ureter.

The bladder and urethra

The bladder and urethra function as a single unit for storage and expulsion of urine, controlled by somatic and autonomic nerves with complex central connections allowing voluntary control over micturition (Fig. 2). Sensory nerves pass primarily in the pelvic parasympathetics (S2–S4) and ascend to micturition centres in the pons via the lateral spinothalamic tracts. Some sensory fibres are sympathetic in origin, passing to the hypogastric plexus, so sacral nerve division does not always abolish bladder sensation completely.

Motor nerves also pass from the pelvic parasympathetics via the *nervi erigentes* to the pelvic ganglia where they are distributed to the detrusor muscle and to the intrinsic urethral sphincter. Sympathetic nerves pass through the same channels but are primarily inhibitory or vasomotor. The rhabdosphincter is innervated by S2–S3 somatic fibres, which travel in the nervi erigentes, while the periurethral muscle sling is supplied by the pudendal nerve.

As the bladder fills, detrusor contractions are inhibited, and continence is maintained by closure of the bladder neck and distal sphincter. A spino-pontine-spinal reflex via the pontine micturition centre plays an important role in coordinating detrusor and sphincter activity, while the anterior part of the frontal lobe produces voluntary inhibition of micturition. Once the bladder becomes full, stretch receptors in the detrusor muscle fire signals via S2–S4 along the lateral spinothalamic tracts to the frontal cortex, and a desire to void is registered. When it is socially appropriate, the frontal cortex facilitates the *micturition reflex*.

As voiding begins, the urethral sphincter relaxes first, together with the pelvic floor and the bladder neck. Parasympathetic activity then initiates a detrusor contraction, which results in the passage of urine; the presence of urine in the urethra produces reflex facilitation of detrusor contraction, which helps to complete voiding. At the end of voiding, these processes are reversed, and the intrinsic muscle of the proximal urethra contracts retrogradely to 'milk back' into the bladder any urine trapped in the urethra. Once all this has taken place, inhibition of the reflex is reapplied by higher centres, and the bladder returns to its resting state.

> ### Key points
>
> ■ The kidney is a complex organ with a high blood flow, which has important homeostatic properties and is able to maintain its function even when tissue perfusion is poor.
>
> ■ The main function of the ureter is peristalsis, which is initiated by pacemaker cells in the minor calyces and results in the progression of a bolus of urine down the ureter due to myogenic propagation.
>
> ■ Reflux of urine is prevented by the nature of the ureterovesical junction, by a 'flutter valve' effect and by ureteric coaption behind each urine bolus.
>
> ■ Storage and evacuation of urine is controlled centrally, and a complex micturition reflex is triggered once the desire to void cannot be resisted and social circumstances permit.

Structure and function of the genital tract

Prostate

Macroscopic structure

The prostate gland surrounds the urethra just below the bladder neck and rests on the pelvic floor muscles. There is little prostate anteriorly, and it is bounded posteriorly by the *fascia of Denonvilliers*; the toughness of this fascia prevents prostatic enlargement or prostate cancer from invading the rectum. The 'true' capsule of the prostate comprises adventitial tissue only, whereas the 'false' (surgical) capsule is a result of compression of the peripheral tissue by benign enlargement of the transition zone. Arterial supply is from the inferior vesical artery, and venous drainage is into an extracapsular plexus of veins that drains with the dorsal penile vein into the iliac vein. Some venous blood drains directly to a plexus of veins in front of the vertebral bodies (*Batson's prevertebral plexus*); this plexus has no valves and explains the tendency of prostate cancer to spread up into the pelvis and spine or down into the femora.

Microscopic structure

The prostate is divided into several lobes (Fig. 1) distinguished by their glandular structure and embryological origin. The secretory glands of the prostate lie in a fibromuscular stroma; the glands of the transition zone (the site of benign enlargement and 10% of tumours) drain via short ducts into the urethra, while the longer glands of the posterior zone (the site of 80% of prostate tumours) enter the urethral sinus close to the prostatic utricle (*verumontanum*).

Physiology

The prostate is a reproductive organ and produces 10–20% of the ejaculate. The stroma has a regulatory function, but the glands produce prostaglandins, sialic acid and acid phosphatase, which play an ill-defined role in fertility; antibacterial agents are also found in prostatic secretions. Prostate growth is driven by *testosterone*, which is metabolised to its active form *dihydrotestosterone* by the enzyme 5-α-reductase; this process is facilitated by prolactin and may be blocked by inhibitory drugs to relieve obstructive urinary symptoms. $α_1$-Adrenergic nerves, which produce muscle constriction, are widely distributed throughout the prostate and may be inhibited by α-blockers to induce smooth muscle relaxation in the prostate.

Vas deferens and seminal vesicle

The vasa deferentia are muscular tubes that arise from the tails of the epididymes and pass upwards along the spermatic cord into the inguinal canal. They enter the pelvis at the internal ring, running along the side-walls before turning medially at the level of the ischial tuberosity. They then become convoluted (*ampullae of the vas deferens*) before joining the seminal vesicles to form the ejaculatory ducts. Each duct pierces the prostate and opens into the floor of the prostatic urethra adjacent to the verumontanum. The seminal vesicles are coiled muscular tubes lying behind the prostate. During orgasm, muscular contractions of the vasa deferentia carry sperm to the ejaculatory duct. The seminal vesicles provide 80% of the ejaculate volume, including nutrients such as fructose. Rhythmic contractions of the vasa and seminal vesicles expel these products during ejaculation and emission of semen.

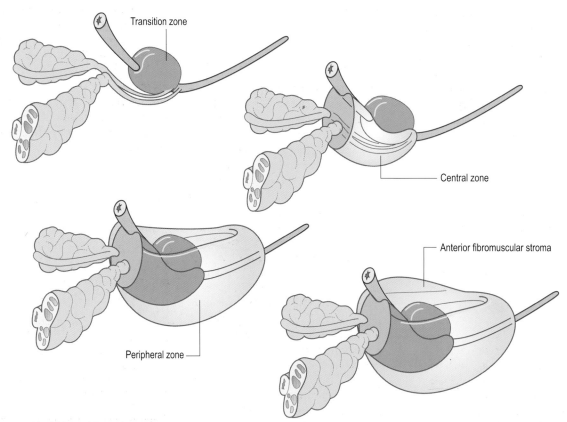

Transition zone

Central zone

Anterior fibromuscular stroma

Peripheral zone

Fig. 1 **Anatomical lobes of the prostate.**

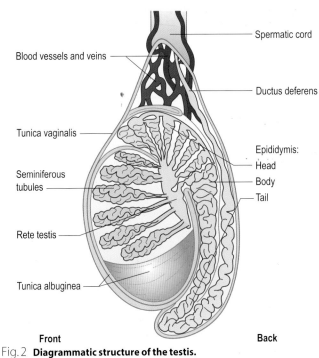

Fig. 2 **Diagrammatic structure of the testis.**

Penis

Macroscopic structure

The penis is composed mainly of two corpora cavernosa that join behind the pubis and form the erectile tissue; proximally, the overlying fascia is fixed to the inferior margin of the pubic bone to form the *suspensory ligament of the penis*. The corpus spongiosum, containing the spongiose urethra, is applied to the ventral surface of the corpora cavernosa and expands distally to form the *glans penis*. Arterial supply is from the external pudendal branch of the femoral artery. Venous drainage is from circumflex veins arising in the corpus spongiosum, emissary veins from the corpora cavernosa and dorsal veins that coalesce to form the dorsal penile vein in front of the prostate. Innervation is by dorsal and cavernous branches from the pudendal nerve.

Microscopic structure

The corpora cavernosa are enclosed by thick fascia (*Buck's fascia*) and contain smooth muscle bundles that form a meshwork of endothelium-lined vascular spaces. These spaces fill with blood to produce erection.

Physiology

Erection is triggered by the cavernous (parasympathetic) nerves, which release acetylcholine and result in local nitric oxide synthesis. This in turn results in activation of cyclic guanosine monophosphate (GMP), which produces smooth muscle relaxation in the corpora cavernosa and an influx of arterial blood. The flow of blood into the penis obstructs the emissary veins, preventing drainage, and an erection results. Detumescence is caused partly by sympathetic vasoconstriction and partly as a result of deactivation of cyclic GMP by the enzyme phosphodiesterase. Inhibitors of phosphodiesterase or injected smooth muscle relaxants (e.g. prostaglandin E1) are used to stimulate erections.

Scrotum

Macroscopic structure

The scrotum is formed of rugose skin, rich in sweat and sebaceous glands; it is incompletely separated into two compartments by a central septum. The subcutaneous (*dartos*) muscle is continuous with Colles' and Scarpa's fascia, which limit expansion of infection or haematomas. Lymphatic drainage is to the superficial inguinal nodes.

Arterial supply is via the testicular artery arising from the abdominal aorta, and venous drainage is into a venous plexus in the spermatic cord (*pampiniform plexus*) and thence into the left testicular vein or the inferior vena cava on the right. Lymphatic drainage follows the arterial supply to para-aortic nodes.

Microscopic structure

Each testis is composed of 600 coiled seminiferous tubules with a basement membrane and several layers of developing germinal cells supported by *Sertoli cells* (Fig. 2). The basal layer consists of spermatogonia, which divide to form primary spermatocytes; these undergo meiotic division to form secondary spermatocytes, maturing into spermatids and, ultimately, spermatozoa. Between the tubules lie interstitial (*Leydig*) cells that are responsible for the majority of testosterone production. The epididymes are coiled tubes that receive spermatozoa via the *vasa efferentia* and expand inferiorly to become the vasa deferentia.

Physiology

Sperm production and testosterone secretion are controlled by feedback loops involving the hypothalamico-pituitary-gonadal axis.

Key points

- The genitalia are anatomically constructed to fulfil specific functions, which are dependent on blood flow, nerve supply and hormone stimulation.
- The fascial layers of the genitalia limit the spread of blood or infection to the spaces enclosed by Scarpa's fascia and Colles' fascia.
- Drug manipulation of genital function is well known to alter erection, sperm production and ejaculation or to produce shrinkage and muscle relaxation of the prostate.

Structure and function of the adrenal glands

Macroscopic structure

The adrenal glands are yellow–brown organs that lie superomedial to the kidneys (Fig. 1) and anterior to the crura of the diaphragm. Unlike the kidneys, the adrenal glands are not contained within the fascia of Gerota, so adrenal haemorrhage is not limited by tamponade within this fascial layer. The right adrenal is pyramidal in shape and lies behind the inferior vena cava (IVC) and the liver. The left adrenal is semilunar and lies behind the pancreas, stomach and spleen (Fig. 2). Medially, the adrenal glands are related to the coeliac ganglia.

Blood supply is by three arteries on each side; the superior adrenal artery arises from the inferior phrenic artery, the middle artery directly from the aorta and the inferior artery from the renal artery. A single adrenal vein drains into the IVC on the right and into the renal vein on the left. Innervation is by autonomic nerves from the coeliac plexus, which predominantly supply the adrenal medulla.

Microscopic structure

Morphologically, each adrenal gland is formed into a central medulla (which produces catecholamines) and a peripheral cortex (which produces steroid hormones). There are three distinct types of cells in the renal cortex: the innermost *zona reticularis*, the middle *zona fasciculata* and the outermost *zona glomerulosa* (Fig. 3). The cells of each zone have specific secretory functions.

Physiology

Adrenal medulla

The adrenal medulla synthesises catecholamines from the amino acid tyrosine in response to any stressful stimulus ('*the fight or flight reaction*'); this stimulus is mediated by sympathetic nerves from the coeliac plexus and is precipitated by factors such as exercise, hypoglycaemia, haemorrhage and emotional distress. Eighty per cent of adrenal catecholamine output is adrenaline, with the remaining 20% being noradrenaline or dopamine.

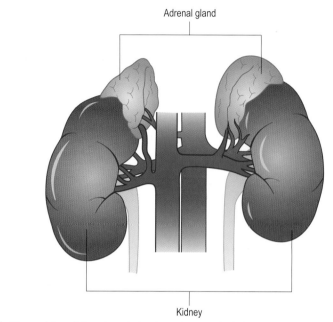

Adrenal gland

Kidney

Fig. 1   **The position of the adrenal glands** in relation to the kidneys.

Table 1 **Systemic effects of humoral catecholamine release**	
Increased cardiac muscle contractility and heart rate	To improve cardiac output
Vasoconstriction	To increase arterial blood pressure
Bronchiolar dilatation	To improve oxygenation
Lipolysis in adipose cells	To aid energy production and preserve glucose reserves
Increased metabolic rate	To increase the ability to move rapidly
Pupillary dilatation	To improve vision under low light conditions
Inhibition of non-essential processes	To shut down processes such as gastrointestinal secretion of gut motility

These are released into the circulation where they exert their effect by binding to adrenergic receptors on target cells.

The effects of humoral catecholamine release by the adrenal glands (Table 1) are identical to those of adrenergic nerve stimulation, but tend to last longer.

Adrenal cortex

The adrenal cortex produces a variety of steroid hormones from the initial substrate cholesterol. Stimulation of the adrenal cortex is brought about by circulating adrenocorticotrophic hormone (ACTH) produced by the anterior pituitary. The zona glomerulosa produces mineralocorticoids (aldosterone), the *zona fasciculata* produces primarily glucocorticoids (e.g. cortisol) and the *zona reticularis* is responsible for sex hormone production.

Aldosterone is produced in response to loss of extracellular fluid volume, high urinary sodium concentrations, hyperkalaemia and activation of the renin–angiotensin system within the

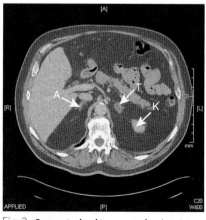

Fig. 2   **Computerised tomography** showing normal right adrenal (A), left adrenal adenoma (T) and normal left kidney (K).

kidney. It works directly on the distal convoluted tubule of the kidney to increase sodium reabsorption and to restore extracellular fluid volume by stimulating transcription of the gene encoding sodium–potassium adenosine triphosphatase (ATPase), thereby increasing the activity of sodium pumps in the tubular epithelial cells.

Glucocorticoids are secreted in response to stimulation by pituitary ACTH, which is released by any form of physical or mental stress; there is a negative feedback mechanism whereby the circulating glucocorticoids prevent further ACTH release by a direct inhibitory action on the hypothalamus and pituitary gland. Glucocorticoids result in gluconeogenesis in the liver, mobilisation of amino acids from tissues, inhibition of glucose uptake by muscle or fat and stimulation of fat breakdown. Glucocorticoids also have potent anti-inflammatory and immunosuppressive properties, which are important in the normal immune response and may be utilised during therapeutic administration. There is a normal diurnal rhythm of ACTH secretion that tends to be highest in the mornings and lowest at night.

Sex hormones (*estrogens, androgens* and *progestogens*) are produced predominantly within the gonads, but a small proportion is produced in the *zona reticularis* of the adrenal cortex. They stimulate the growth of hormone-dependent cells in the genital tract and are responsible to a minor degree for normal sexual development, as well as for some pathological processes such as benign prostatic hyperplasia.

performed extraperitoneally via a loin approach (through the bed of the 11th or 12th rib). The incision is made along the line of the rib, dividing the serratus posterior inferior muscle and the latissimus dorsi; the rib is usually resected or elevated from its periosteum, taking care not to damage the underlying pleural cavity. Once the lumbodorsal fascia is divided deep to the rib, the perirenal fascia is easily identified and the adrenal gland exposed on the superomedial border of the kidney. Large adrenal tumours may require wider exposure than that offered by a loin incision and are best approached through a thoracoabdominal incision with division of the diaphragm down to the adrenal gland. Bilateral adrenalectomy is best performed via a transperitoneal upper abdominal incision.

Technically, the right adrenal is more difficult to access surgically because it tends to lie behind the IVC. It is also technically more difficult to excise because the right adrenal vein is often very short and easily torn during surgery. The left adrenal vein is particularly prone to damage during clamping of the neck of a leaking abdominal aortic aneurysm, which often lies directly behind the left renal vein.

The rich blood supply of the adrenal glands means that they are often the site of metastatic disease, especially from primary tumours of the bronchus, breast, stomach, colon, kidney and bile ducts. Ten per cent of all patients with malignancy undergoing post-mortem examination are found to have adrenal metastases.

Surgery and the adrenal gland

Most urologists now prefer a laparoscopic approach to the adrenal gland (either extraperitoneal or transperitoneal) with significant reduction in morbidity, mortality and hospital stay. Open surgical exposure of the adrenal gland is usually

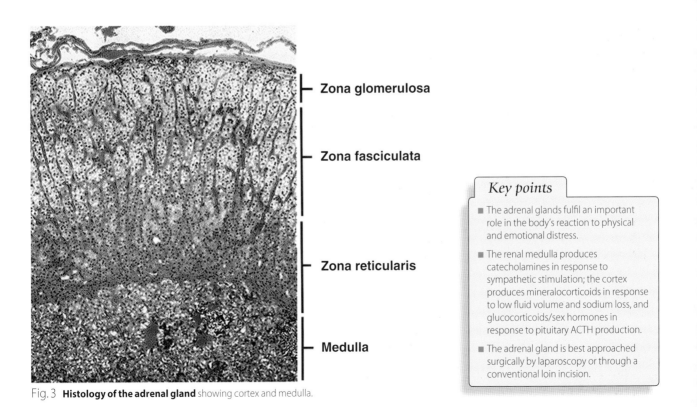

Fig. 3 **Histology of the adrenal gland** showing cortex and medulla.

— Zona glomerulosa

— Zona fasciculata

— Zona reticularis

— Medulla

Key points

■ The adrenal glands fulfil an important role in the body's reaction to physical and emotional distress.

■ The renal medulla produces catecholamines in response to sympathetic stimulation; the cortex produces mineralocorticoids in response to low fluid volume and sodium loss, and glucocorticoids/sex hormones in response to pituitary ACTH production.

■ The adrenal gland is best approached surgically by laparoscopy or through a conventional loin incision.

Investigating the Urological Patient

Taking a urological history

A well-taken history is the starting point for the diagnosis and treatment of all urological patients. The primary symptom complex, the past medical history and the family history give important pointers to the direction that investigation and management should take.

The primary symptom complex

Many patients have multiple symptoms, and recognising the pattern of these symptoms is important in determining the appropriate investigation and management. In all patients, it is important to determine:

- How long have the symptoms been present?
- How severe are the symptoms?
- Do the symptoms vary in severity?
- How much do the symptoms interfere with daily living?

Some symptoms can be assessed using specific questionnaires (Table 1). Questionnaires should be an adjunct or introduction to a detailed urological history and not a substitute for talking to patients. Patients should be allowed to explain symptoms in their own terms, but may need to be guided towards answering specific questions relating to the primary symptom complex.

Pain in the genitourinary tract

Pain is usually due to inflammation or obstruction in the urinary tract.

- *Renal pain* starts in the costovertebral angle and radiates into the hypochondrium or epigastrium. Inflammatory renal pain is usually constant whereas the pain of obstruction tends to wax and wane. Patients often demonstrate renal pain with a typical hand gesture. Similar pain may be seen with musculoskeletal, myofascial or ligamentous inflammation.
- *Ureteric pain* is similar to renal pain but is usually due to obstruction. If the obstruction moves, as it does with a ureteric calculus, the pain moves from flank to iliac fossa, groin and even the scrotum or labia. The site of the pain may help in determining the level of obstruction.
- *Bladder pain* is usually due to obstruction (acute retention) or inflammation of the bladder wall. Inflammatory conditions produce pain that worsens with bladder filling, and there may be severe pain at completion of voiding (strangury). Associated irritative urinary symptoms are common. Bladder pain is often referred to the distal urethra, and pain after voiding suggests an origin from the prostate, the para-urethral glands or the urethra itself.
- *Prostatic pain* is poorly localised and is felt in the lower abdomen, groins, scrotum, lower back, perineum or rectum. It is often associated with lower urinary tract symptoms (LUTS) or erectile dysfunction.
- *Penile pain* is usually due to inflammation in the bladder, prostate or urethra, but may also be caused by preputial problems. Pain in the erect penis is usually due to Peyronie's disease or to priapism.
- *Scrotal pain* may arise from the scrotal contents and from the scrotal wall, or may be referred from higher in the

Table 1 **Examples of symptom questionnaires in urology (see Appendix)**	
Primary symptom complex	**Questionnaire**
Lower urinary tract symptoms	International Prostate Symptom Score (I-PSS)
Bladder pain	Interstitial Cystitis (IC) Symptom Score
Erectile dysfunction	International Index of Erectile Function (IIEF)
Chronic prostatic (pelvic) pain	National Institute of Health Chronic Prostatitis Symptom Index (NIH-CPSI)

urinary tract. Aching pain in the left testis, which improves on lying down, is typical of a varicocele.

Blood in the urine

Gross haematuria is more likely to be associated with significant pathology than microscopic haematuria, but both should be fully evaluated. Initial haematuria usually arises from the prostate or urethra whereas total haematuria suggests an origin in the bladder or upper tracts. Terminal haematuria is usually due to inflammation of the bladder neck or prostate.

Blood clots often accompany haematuria and can cause clot retention (bladder pain). Worm-like clots originate in the upper urinary tract and are shaped by their passage down the ureter. The association of pain with blood in the urine suggests an inflammatory condition, whereas bleeding due to urothelial malignancy is usually painless.

Lower urinary tract symptoms (LUTS)

LUTS may be primarily irritative, obstructive or a combination of both (Table 2). The International Prostate Symptom Score (I-PSS; see Appendix, p. 151) is designed for the assessment of LUTS and is used not only for diagnosis but also to monitor symptom response to treatment.

Incontinence of urine

This is the involuntary loss of urine from the urethra. The commonest pattern is a mixture of stress and urge incontinence in women.

- *Continuous incontinence* is usually due to an ectopic ureter or a urinary fistula.
- *Stress incontinence* is leakage during straining; it is most commonly seen in women after multiple childbirth and in men following prostatic surgery.
- *Urge incontinence* is the sudden loss of urine after an urgent desire to void. It is most commonly due to inflammatory disorders of the bladder or to detrusor instability.
- *Overflow incontinence* is usually the result of chronic (painless) retention of urine.
- *Nocturnal enuresis* in adults is usually due to chronic retention of urine. In children, it improves with maturation of the central nervous system but persists in 15% by the age of 5 years and in 1% by the age of 15 years.
- *Post-micturition dribbling* occurs a few minutes after voiding, usually in young men, and should not be confused with terminal dribbling due to obstructive LUTS.

Sexual dysfunction (see pp. 142 and 143)

Blood in the semen (haematospermia)

This is usually due to low-grade inflammation in the prostate or seminal vesicles and may be associated with prostatic pain.

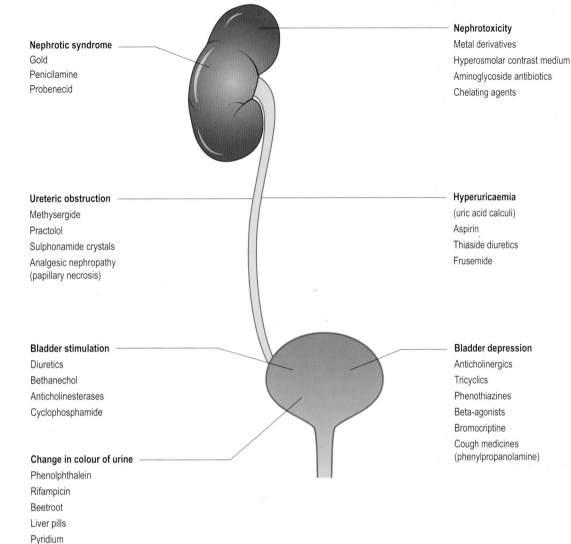

Nephrotoxicity
Metal derivatives
Hyperosmolar contrast medium
Aminoglycoside antibiotics
Chelating agents

Nephrotic syndrome
Gold
Penicilamine
Probenecid

Ureteric obstruction
Methysergide
Practolol
Sulphonamide crystals
Analgesic nephropathy
(papillary necrosis)

Hyperuricaemia
(uric acid calculi)
Aspirin
Thiaside diuretics
Frusemide

Bladder stimulation
Diuretics
Bethanechol
Anticholinesterases
Cyclophosphamide

Bladder depression
Anticholinergics
Tricyclics
Phenothiazines
Beta-agonists
Bromocriptine
Cough medicines
(phenylpropanolamine)

Change in colour of urine
Phenolphthalein
Rifampicin
Beetroot
Liver pills
Pyridium

Fig. 1 **Diseases and treatments that may affect the urinary tract.**

Table 2 **Lower urinary tract symptoms (LUTS)**	
Obstructive	**Irritative**
Delay in initiating micturition (hesitancy)	Daytime frequency
Reduction in strength of the urinary stream	Nocturia
Stopping and starting (intermittency)	Urgency
Dribbling at completion (terminal dribbling)	Urge incontinence
Straining to void	Pain on voiding (dysuria)
Sense of incomplete bladder emptying	

It normally settles within a few weeks and does not require investigation unless prostate cancer is suspected clinically.

Gas bubbles in the urine (pneumaturia)

This is caused by either urinary infection with a gas-forming organism or a fistula between the bowel and the urinary tract. It is often associated with other urinary symptoms and with bowel symptoms.

Urethral discharge (see pp. 38 and 39)

Past medical history

Many urological patients are elderly and have chronic, multi-system diseases that not only cause urological problems but also influence decisions about the medical or surgical treatment of their condition. The urinary tract can be affected by many diseases and also by their treatment (Fig. 1). For example, diabetes mellitus or multiple sclerosis often produce LUTS, and hypertension or its treatment may produce erectile dysfunction. A full history of previous operations, including those involving the urinary tract, is important in obtaining an accurate picture of the patient's symptoms. All patients should be asked about smoking (which causes urothelial malignancy and erectile dysfunction), alcohol consumption and current medications.

Key points

- A carefully taken history provides the foundation for the assessment of all urological symptoms and sets the tone for the relationship between clinician and patient.

- Specific symptom scoring systems are a useful introduction to any discussion of urological symptoms but cannot replace a well-taken history.

- Recognition of specific symptom patterns helps to determine both the nature of the underlying problem and the direction of future investigations.

- Many urological patients are elderly and have multisystem diseases or are taking medications that may affect the urinary tract.

- Many urological conditions have a familial or genetic basis, which may be relevant in risk assessment and further management.

Examination of the urological patient

Physical examination often reveals few clinical signs in the urological patient, but a careful general examination and assessment of the urological system may reveal subtle abnormalities.

General examination

General examination of the patient starts with determining whether s/he appears well or ill. This includes assessment of general body habitus, nutritional status, cachexia, anaemia, jaundice, skin colour and lymphadenopathy. Peripheral oedema may indicate hypoproteinaemia, venous/lymphatic obstruction, cardiac failure, chronic renal failure or nephrotic syndrome. The site of any abdominal mass should be recorded together with areas of localised tenderness and guarding; gentle percussion is a kinder means of eliciting local peritonism than eliciting rebound tenderness.

A full neurological assessment is essential in patients with lower urinary tract symptoms (LUTS) or erectile dysfunction, and assessment of the sacral reflexes is an essential part of this assessment (Fig. 1). The bladder and penis are innervated primarily by the S2, S3 and S4 nerve roots, and assessment of the bulbospongiosus reflex in particular has been termed 'the urologist's knee jerk'.

The peripheral pulses should be palpated, especially in the lower limbs; the blood pressure should be measured and a full assessment made of the heart and lungs by percussion and auscultation. The breasts should be examined for gynaecomastia, which may be seen in endocrine disease, liver failure, exogenous administration of antiandrogens for prostate cancer or estrogen production by a testicular tumour.

Urological examination

Kidneys

The kidneys are not normally palpable in the upper abdomen, but the lower pole of a normal right kidney may be palpable in children and thin women on deep inspiration; the right kidney is more readily felt because it is displaced caudally by the liver. Any mass arising in the loin should be palpated bimanually to differentiate between hepatic or splenic enlargement and a palpable kidney. Loin tenderness is detected by gentle percussion in the loin. Renal artery stenosis, aortic aneurysms and a renal arteriovenous fistula may produce an audible bruit, heard with a stethoscope placed in the epigastrium. The skin of the loin and upper abdomen may show the typical vesicles of herpes zoster in patients with loin pain, while the spine and paravertebral muscles should be examined to exclude nerve root (T10–L1) irritation; this may be associated with reduced sensation or hyperaesthesia in the loin.

Bladder

The bladder cannot be percussed or palpated above the symphysis pubis unless it contains more than 150 mL of urine. The finding of suprapubic dullness to percussion is particularly useful if the patient has just passed urine. The presence of significant residual urine can be confirmed by ultrasound scanning of the lower abdomen using a simple, hand-held scanner that measures bladder volume. Tenderness over the

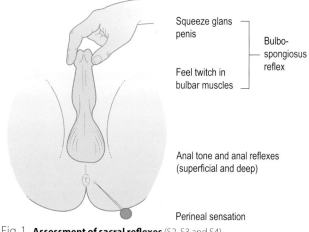

Fig. 1 **Assessment of sacral reflexes** (S2, S3 and S4).

Squeeze glans penis
Feel twitch in bulbar muscles
Bulbo-spongiosus reflex
Anal tone and anal reflexes (superficial and deep)
Perineal sensation

bladder indicates inflammation but, if the bladder is enlarged and acutely tender, this is characteristic of acute retention of urine. The enlarged bladder of chronic retention of urine is usually painless and non-tender. An enlarged bladder does not always appear as a midline structure so even an asymmetric mass arising from the pelvis may be an enlarged bladder; ultimately, ultrasound or catheterisation may be required to determine whether a pelvic mass is an enlarged bladder.

Groins

The hernial orifices are assessed with the patient both lying and standing. An inguinal hernia arises above and lateral to the pubic tubercle whereas a femoral hernia arises below and lateral to the tubercle. Coughing, straining or a Valsalva manoeuvre will usually make a hernia more obvious. Small inguinal hernias can impinge on the ilioinguinal nerve (L1) and cause inguinoscrotal pain.

Penis

The penis should be felt between the fingers for any abnormal areas of thickening and palpated along the ventral aspect to reveal thickening or tenderness along the line of the urethra. The position of the urethral meatus should be noted, together with any reddening of the orifice, which might suggest urethritis. Any abnormality of the foreskin or scarring and shortening of the penile frenulum should be assessed. In adults or children with an abnormally placed ventral meatus (hypospadias), the foreskin is often incomplete ventrally and has a hooded appearance (Fig. 2). In uncircumcised men, the

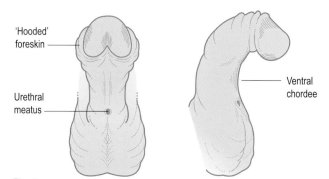

'Hooded' foreskin
Urethral meatus
Ventral chordee

Fig. 2 **Hypospadias** with an associated hooded prepuce.

foreskin should be gently retracted to expose the glans penis and coronal sulcus. The penile skin, including the glans penis, may itself show ulceration, changes of balanitis xerotica obliterans, venereal warts or collections of vesicles due to herpes simplex.

Scrotum

The scrotal wall is examined for any visible or palpable abnormality. Small angiokeratomas on the scrotal skin are common and of no clinical significance (Fig. 3). The scrotal contents must be assessed in a systematic manner with sequential palpation of each spermatic cord, vas deferens, epididymis and testis. The shape, size and consistency of any swelling should be recorded and its relationship to the underlying structures carefully assessed. If it is possible to get above the swelling in the scrotum, it arises from the scrotal contents and is a true scrotal swelling; if it is not possible to get above a scrotal swelling, it is most likely that the swelling is arising from the groin and is an indirect inguinal hernia. True scrotal swellings should be characterised into solid, inflammatory or cystic. Inflammatory swellings show all the signs of inflammation (heat, redness and pain). The hallmarks of cystic swellings are fluctuation on two planes, and most cystic swellings transilluminate provided a strong enough source of light is used. A swelling above the left testis that feels like a 'bag of worms' is probably a varicocele; varicoceles become more obvious when the patient stands, coughs or performs a Valsalva manoeuvre and are seen on the left side in 98% of cases. The sudden development of a left-sided varicocele suggests a left renal tumour, and varicoceles on the right are often associated with retroperitoneal tumours.

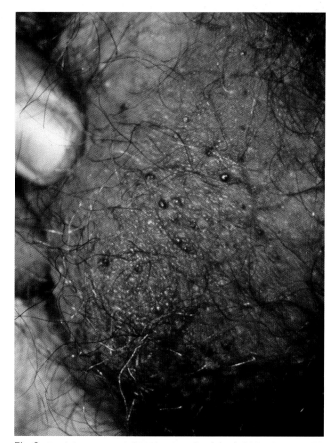

Fig. 3 **Angiokeratomas (of Fordyce) on the scrotal skin.**

Prostate

Digital rectal examination, performed with the patient in the left lateral position, forms an important part of urological assessment. The normal prostate weighs approximately 15 g, is the size of a chestnut and has the same texture as the tip of the nose. Any firmness, tenderness, induration or nodularity should be noted together with the mobility of the rectal mucosa over the prostate. The actual size of the prostate has no bearing on the severity of symptoms caused by the prostate, and an enlarged bladder can make the prostate feel larger than it really is by pushing it downwards and backwards into the rectal lumen. Seventy per cent of prostate cancers arise in the posterior zone of the prostate and are palpable via the rectum, whereas 25% of rectal cancers are also within reach of the palpating finger. It may be possible to feel the seminal vesicles,

above and lateral to the prostate, especially if they are enlarged or inflamed.

Female pelvis

The female pelvis is examined systematically in a position that is comfortable for the patient. The external genitalia, introitus and urethra should be clearly visible, and an assessment can be made of estrogenisation in these areas. Asking the patient to cough may reveal anterior or posterior vaginal prolapse, together with stress incontinence. The urethra can be palpated along the anterior vaginal wall and, finally, an assessment can be made of the uterus, adnexa and fornices by bimanual palpation. A stone in the lower ureter may occasionally be palpable in the lateral fornix of the vagina.

> *Key points*
>
> - A careful, general examination of all body systems is important in the assessment of urological symptoms.
>
> - Specific attention should be directed to each individual area of the genitourinary tract, and these should all be examined in a systematic fashion.
>
> - Rectal examination in males and pelvic assessment in females are essential, especially in the assessment of lower urinary tract symptoms.

Laboratory investigations

Urine examination

Simple urinalysis

Urine is usually tested using a dipstick, which measures specific characteristics of the urine (Table 1, Fig. 1). The presence of glycosuria suggests diabetes mellitus or a low renal threshold for glucose, and should be investigated further with a fasting blood sugar or a formal glucose tolerance test.

Low specific gravity (<1008) suggests chronic renal failure, high fluid intake, polyuria or inappropriate antidiuretic hormone (ADH) secretion. High specific gravity (>1020) is caused by dehydration or administration of intravenous contrast medium.

Dip testing detects more than five red blood cells per microlitre. More than two blood cells suggests a high risk of urothelial cancer and should prompt full investigations; lower levels of red blood cells in the urine can be investigated in a more limited manner. Anticoagulation at normal therapeutic levels does not result in a positive urine test for blood.

Normal urine pH is between 4.5 and 8.0. Higher levels (>7.5) suggest the presence of a urease-splitting organism (*Proteus vulgaris*). pH <4.5 is suggestive of high uric acid levels.

Protein levels of more than 0.3 g/L are detected by dipstick. If persistent proteinuria is found, more detailed quantification is necessary from a 24-h urine collection.

Nitrates and leucocytes in the urine suggest the presence of infection. The persistence of leucocytes in sterile urine (*sterile pyuria*) is usually due to incompletely treated urinary infection, urothelial malignancy or stone disease and only rarely to tuberculosis.

Microscopy

Urine microscopy may show red blood cells, white blood cells, epithelial cells, casts (Fig. 2), crystals, yeasts, bacteria and parasitic ova. Normal urine contains less than three red blood cells per high-powered field (HPF). Glomerular red cells tend to be large and dysmorphic, whereas red cells from the lower urinary tract are usually eumorphic. Cellular casts suggest glomerular disease. Oxalate, urate and cystine crystals may be seen in acidic urine (pH <5.5), while phosphate crystallises in alkaline urine (pH >6.0). Significant bacteriuria is defined as five organisms per HPF and equates to colony counts of 100 000/mL.

Culture and sensitivity

Urine for culture and sensitivity is usually collected as a midstream or catheter specimen, but suprapubic aspiration is sometimes used in infants. Urine should be cultured within 1 h of production or refrigerated at 5°C. The presence of >100 000 organisms/mL confirms a significant urinary infection, whereas levels of <10 000/mL suggest contamination. If organisms are cultured from the urine, Gram staining is performed to identify the organisms and assess antibiotic sensitivity. Yeasts (e.g.

Candida albicans) may also be cultured from the urine in susceptible individuals. If tuberculosis is suspected, three early-morning urine samples (EMUs) should be submitted for culture (on *Lowenstein–Jensen medium*) and specific bacteriological staining (*Ziehl–Neelsen*).

Biochemistry

Biochemical analysis of the urine is needed in stone patients (Table 2). Persistent proteinuria is an indication for more detailed quantification in a 24-h urine collection.

Cystological examination

In suspected urothelial malignancy or in those patients being followed for transitional cell tumours, cytological examination of the urine is essential. A freshly voided specimen is collected and centrifuged to retrieve the cell-containing sediment; the sediment is then resuspended, treated with *Papanicolaou stain* and examined carefully for malignant cells.

Tumour markers

Special assays are being developed to detect malignant cells in the urine (e.g. bladder tumour antigen, minichromosome maintenance protein type 5); such tests are not routinely used and remain under experimental assessment.

Table 1 Parameters assessed by dipstick urinalysis
Glucose
Bilirubin
Ketones
Specific gravity
Blood
pH
Protein
Urobilinogen
Nitrates
Leucocytes

Table 2 Urine biochemical investigations in suspected stone formers
Osmolarity
Electrolytes (sodium, potassium)
Creatinine
Uric acid
Oxalate
Calcium and phosphorus
Citrate
Amino acid screen

Blood tests

Biochemistry

Blood tests should be tailored to the individual patient and to the primary symptom complex (Table 3). Simple tests of renal function (electrolytes, urea and creatinine) are indicated for most patients, but are insensitive indicators of impaired renal function. Prostate-specific

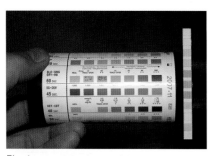

Fig. 1 **Dipstick urine testing.**

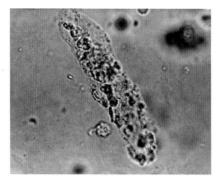

Fig. 2 **Tubular casts in the urine.**

Table 3 **Indications for specific blood tests**	
Diagnosis	**Investigations**
Renal failure (acute/chronic)	Autoantibodies
	Complement levels
	Immunoglobulins
	Osmolarity
	Aluminium/magnesium levels
Stone disease	Plasma urate
	Bone function
	Parathyroid hormone
Suspected liver disease	Liver function tests
Suspected adrenal tumour	Cortisol
	Adrenocorticotrophic hormone
	Catecholamines
Infertility/erectile dysfunction	Follicle-stimulating hormone, luteinising hormone and thyroid-stimulating hormone
	Testosterone and prolactin
Suspected renal tumour	Liver function tests
	Bone function tests
	Parathyroid hormone/erythropoietin
Lower urinary tract symptoms	Prostate-specific antigen
Suspected/known prostate cancer	Alkaline phosphatase
Urinary diversion	Chloride
	Creatinine clearance

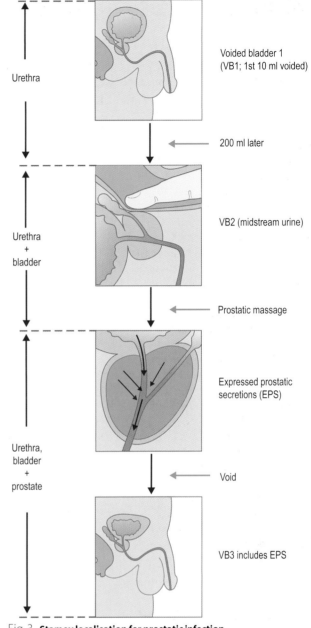

Fig. 3 **Stamey localisation for prostatic infection.**

antigen (PSA) measurement is indicated in men under the age of 70 years with lower urinary tract symptoms, and levels should be interpreted according to age (see p. 126).

Haematology

A full blood count may detect anaemia, polycythaemia and white cell abnormalities (e.g. leucocytosis). Erythrocyte sedimentation rate (ESR) is rarely measured routinely but is helpful in the follow-up of idiopathic retroperitoneal fibrosis. Patients of Afro-Caribbean descent should undergo screening for sickle cell disease before anaesthesia. Patients taking anticoagulants or those with clotting disorders should undergo formal assessment of their coagulation. Blood grouping and cross-matching is necessary for patients who may require a blood transfusion for anaemia or during urological surgery.

Serology

Specific serological investigation may be indicated in patients with sexually transmitted disease (see pp. 38 and 39).

Semen analysis (see pp. 144 and 145)

Localisation of infection

Stamey localisation for prostatic infection

In patients with suspected chronic prostatic infection, a Stamey localisation test (Fig. 3) may help to characterise the type and site of infection.

Two-glass test for urethritis (see pp. 38 and 39)

Key points

- Urinalysis using a proprietary dipstick detects abnormalities in the urine, which may point to a specific diagnosis and direct further investigations.

- Suspected urinary infection should be confirmed by the finding of > 100 000 organisms/mL urine on bacteriological culture.

- Biochemical tests on blood and urine should not be requested blindly, but should be tailored to an individual symptom complex or suspected diagnosis.

- Simple infection-localising tests are helpful in men with urethritis or prostatitis.

Ultrasound in urology

Ultrasound is simple, cheap, safe and effective in evaluating a wide variety of urological problems (Table 1) and avoiding the risks of radiation exposure. It provides good anatomical and physiological information, can be performed at the bedside and is especially useful in assessing infants or children who are uncooperative.

Ultrasound physics

Pulses of high-frequency sound waves entering the body are reflected, refracted or absorbed by the tissues depending on the nature of those tissues. The ultrasound transducer also acts as a receiver for reflected signals, which are displayed visually in real time. The time taken for the echoes to return to the transducer is a measure of the distance of the organ from the transducer. Most ultrasound transducers can be orientated to produce images in virtually any anatomical plane. Transducer frequency varies from 3.5 to 15 MHz; higher frequencies generally produce greater resolution but less tissue penetration.

Ultrasound may be hampered by body fat, bowel gas or bony landmarks such as ribs, and is not helpful in the assessment of areas such as the retroperitoneum or intra-abdominal ureter. To some extent, the quality of information obtained is only as good as the ultrasonographer.

Greyscale imaging
This is the mainstay of real-time, two-dimensional ultrasound. Fluid-filled lesions demonstrate anechoic centres with clearly visible walls and distal sound enhancement. Solid lesions demonstrate internal echoes whose appearances may be typical of specific abnormalities (e.g. the high echogenicity of fat in a renal angiomyolipoma or the whorled appearance of a testicular epidermoid cyst).

Doppler blood flow imaging
This is often used as an adjunct to greyscale imaging to observe the strength and direction of blood flow. Duplex scanning permits the measurement of vascular waveforms and allows a colour-coded signal representing blood flow to be superimposed on the greyscale image. Doppler imaging is particularly useful in assessing transplant kidneys, renal trauma, solid masses in the upper tracts and scrotal swellings where vascular assessment is important (e.g. varicoceles and suspected torsion of the testis).

Use of contrast agents or bubbles in the urinary tract
The use of contrast medium in ultrasound remains under assessment for investigating the renal vasculature. Bubble ultrasound has been used experimentally to detect ureteric reflux of bubble-laden fluid instilled into the bladder.

Three-dimensional imaging
This complex technology is in its infancy but permits reconstruction of an organ from a series of greyscale slices. It has potential in the assessment of small, focal lesions in specific organs and has been used experimentally in the assessment of prostate cancer.

Table 1 **Main indications for ultrasound in urology**
Renal parenchymal abnormalities (masses and cysts)
Renal calculi
Upper tract obstruction
Recurrent urinary infection
Bladder abnormalities
Prostatic abnormalities and biopsy
Scrotal swellings
Blood flow measurement
Penile and urethral problems
Abscesses and fluid collections
Renal trauma

Ultrasound-guided biopsy
Biopsy attachments allow samples to be taken from localised lesions under direct vision with great accuracy. The technique can be used in any organ but is most widely employed for renal masses, for enlarged lymph nodes and in the prostate. The use of very fine needles means that the potential for tumour seeding in biopsy tracts is minimal.

Ultrasound of the kidneys and bladder

This forms the mainstay of urological imaging for patients with recurrent urinary tract infections, lower urinary tract symptoms (LUTS), renal calculi, suspected upper tract masses and for those patients with haematuria with a low risk of malignancy (age less than 45 years, non-smokers, no chemical exposure or less than 2+ of microhaematuria). Ultrasound gives good information about parenchymal texture and space-occupying lesions, including cysts or solid masses, and demonstrates the anatomy of the collecting system. It cannot reliably resolve lesions that are less than 5 mm in diameter and provides little information about function other than confirming that blood flow is present.

The normal ureter cannot be visualised using ultrasound, but dilatation of the lower ureter may be seen, especially just behind the bladder. Bladder wall thickness, filling defects (Fig. 1), diverticula, ureteroceles, foreign bodies and bladder

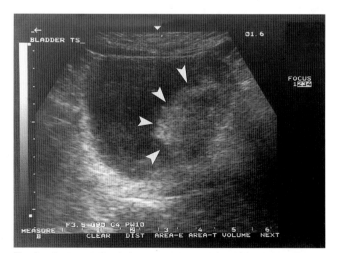

Fig. 1 **Bladder ultrasound** showing a superficial bladder tumour.

calculi can all be detected with ultrasound, and post-micturition residual urine can be computed by measuring the bladder in three dimensions. Some cheaper ultrasound systems are available that do not produce images but simply give a computation of bladder volume; these are useful at the bedside to determine the effectiveness of bladder emptying after catheter removal, after bladder neck surgery or during the assessment of LUTS. Ultrasound-guided puncture of the balloon is the optimum method for removing a self-retaining catheter that will not deflate.

Ultrasound of the prostate

The prostate can be seen by abdominal ultrasound but is best visualised using a transrectal transducer. Transrectal ultrasound (Fig. 2) is the investigation of choice for imaging the prostate, and this technique is particularly useful in assessing men with suspected prostate cancer. Prostatic volume and prostate-specific antigen (PSA) density (PSA level/prostatic volume) can be measured and specific anatomical zones of the prostate can be biopsied systematically using a transducer that scans in both transverse and longitudinal planes. The seminal vesicles and ejaculatory ducts can also be visualised in men with obstructive infertility or obstructed ejaculation.

Ultrasound of the scrotum

Ultrasound is ideal for assessing scrotal swellings and blood flow in the spermatic cord or testis. Swellings that may be difficult to feel through the scrotal wall can be demonstrated with ease, and solid masses can be localised anatomically; masses in the body of the testis are invariably malignant whereas extratesticular masses are usually benign.

Ultrasound of the urethra and penis

Ultrasound of the penis has limited use other than in the assessment of penile blood flow in erectile dysfunction. Ultrasound of the urethra is not widely used, but studies during voiding can produce clear information about urethral strictures (Fig. 3), diverticula, venereal warts and valves without the need for urethral catheterisation, urethroscopy or contrast administration. It also gives information about periurethral fibrosis, which helps in deciding the best treatment for urethral strictures.

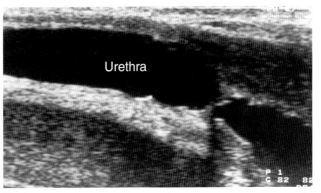

Fig. 3 **Ultrasound urethrogram** of a strictured urethra.

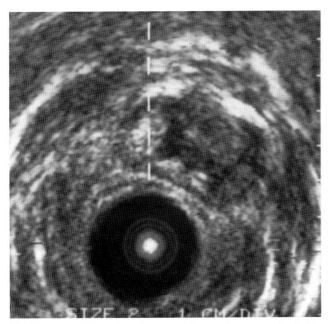

Fig. 2 **Transrectal prostatic ultrasound** showing the computerised grid used for guiding prostatic biopsy.

Key points

- Ultrasound is simple, safe, cheap and avoids the risks of ionising radiation.
- It is the main investigation for the commonest conditions in urology (lower urinary tract symptoms, recurrent urinary infections and haematuria), although further imaging techniques may be needed if abnormalities are found.
- Little functional information can be obtained with ultrasound, apart from measurement of blood flow.
- Transrectal ultrasound is the investigation of choice to obtain biopsy material in men with suspected prostate cancer.
- Other ultrasound techniques (urethral scanning, contrast ultrasound and three-dimensional reconstruction) are still under development.

The intravenous urogram

The intravenous urogram (IVU) provides anatomical information as well as a degree of functional information, but is now used less often because of advances in other forms of imaging.

There are now few indications for an IVU (Table 1). Specific protocols are normally used; in suspected renal colic, a plain radiograph with 5-min and 20-min post-injection films is required. Every IVU needs to be tailored to the abnormalities noted as the examination progresses.

The plain abdominal radiograph (KUB)

The preliminary plain film should include the full length of the abdomen from kidneys to urethra; occasionally, more than one film may be needed to include all these structures. It shows calcific opacities, anatomical landmarks, soft tissues, intestinal gas pattern and any skeletal abnormalities.

Calcific opacities

Ninety per cent of stones in the urinary tract are radio-opaque but may not be visible once contrast medium has been given unless a plain film is performed first. Only 50% of ureteric calculi are recognised as such on the KUB, and calcific opacities (Fig. 1) may not be in the urinary tract. Radiodense opacities in the pelvic area are usually calcifications

Table 1   **Indications for IVU**
Renal or ureteric pain
Suspected upper tract stones
Suspected ureteric injury (usually post-operative)
Congenital upper tract abnormalities
Renovascular disease
Ureteric localisation prior to radical pelvic surgery

in pelvic veins (phleboliths); these are circular and have a central 'hole' formed by the lumen of the vein.

Organ outlines

The outlines of liver, kidneys, spleen and bladder are often visible on the KUB (Fig. 2). The psoas muscles, the retroperitoneal fat pad ('flank stripe') and soft-tissue masses can usually be identified on the KUB. The bowel gas pattern may suggest intestinal disease, and an erect film may show fluid levels or free intraperitoneal air. Calcification in the wall of an abdominal aortic aneurysm or other blood vessels may also be seen on the KUB. Calcification of the vas deferens is often seen in diabetic patients.

Bony abnormalities

Musculoskeletal abnormalities such as spinal dysraphism or sacral agenesis can

be identified on the KUB. Bony metastases may be seen anywhere in the skeleton and may give rise to visible pathological fractures. Sclerotic metastases from carcinoma of the prostate are usually seen in the axial skeleton (spine, pelvis and upper femora).

Administration of contrast medium

Contrast medium (50–100 mL) is normally administered as a rapid intravenous bolus. Most contrast medium is hyperosmolar (1400–2400 Osm/kg water), but the newer, non-ionic agents have reduced osmolarity and a reduced risk of adverse reactions (Table 2).

Adverse contrast reactions

These are due to either direct chemotoxicity or anaphylaxis. They are more likely in patients with dehydration, chronic renal failure, multiple myeloma, a history of atopy and in diabetics taking oral metformin. Pretreatment with steroids and avoidance of dehydration may reduce the risk of an adverse

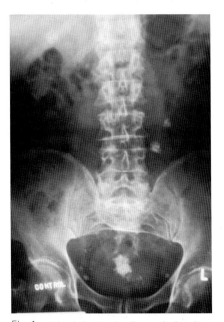

Fig. 1   **Plain abdominal radiograph showing multiple calcific opacities.**

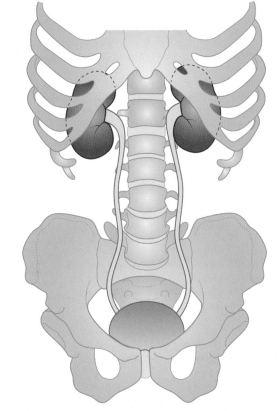

Fig. 2   **Landmarks of the urinary tract on the KUB.**

Table 2 **Adverse reactions to intravenous contrast medium**		
Adverse reaction	**High-osmolarity agents**	**Low-osmolarity agents**

Minor
  Nausea
  Flushing
  Heat
	10%	3.5%

Intermediate
  Vomiting
  Itching
  Facial flushing
	3%	1%

Nephrotoxicity	0.15%	0.15%

Severe
  Urticaria
  Facial oedema
  Laryngeal oedema
  Bronchospasm
	0.3%	0.09%

Fatal	1 in 230 000	1 in 350 000

reaction, and metformin should be stopped for 48 h before giving intravenous contrast medium.

The nephrogram phase

Films taken within the first 2–3 min are useful for showing mass lesions, renal scarring or poor vascularisation of the kidneys. Nephrotomography may help in the assessment of mass lesions in the kidney.

A persistent faint nephrogram suggests glomerulonephritis or acute tubular necrosis, while increasingly dense or longlasting nephrograms are seen with obstruction of the ureter and chronic renal artery stenosis respectively. Pools of contrast medium in dilated calyces suggest obstruction or non-obstructive dilatation of the kidneys.

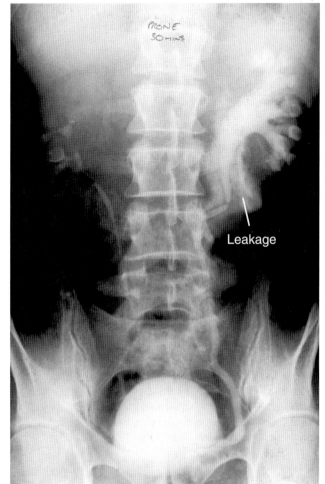

Fig. 3 **Extravasation of contrast from the left kidney due to stone obstruction in the ureter.**

The pyelogram phase

Five minutes after injection, excretion of the contrast medium into the collecting system usually begins. Filling defects in the collecting system or ureters may be seen, and specifically targeted films or tomograms may be necessary in this situation. Acute obstruction of the ureter may be associated with rupture of a papillary fornix and extravasation of contrast medium (Fig. 3). Chronic obstruction (e.g. pelviureteric junction obstruction) cannot easily be differentiated from non-obstructive dilatation, but a supplementary intravenous dose of diuretic causes obstructed systems to increase in size while atonically dilated systems clear the contrast medium.

Table 3 **Follow-up of abnormalities detected by IVU**	
Abnormality	**Next diagnostic step**
Possible absent kidney	Ultrasound or computerised tomography (CT)
Obstruction	Ultrasound, retrograde pyelography or CT
Mass	CT or ultrasound
Vascular compromise	Radionuclide scintigraphy
Renal scarring	Radionuclide scintigraphy or ultrasound
Previous nephrectomy	Patient history

Special films

Oblique views of the ureter may help in localising calcifications, prone films may encourage drainage of dilated unobstructed kidneys, delayed films may reveal the site of ureteric obstruction if the ureter is not well seen, and a post-micturition film may help to assess bladder emptying.

Follow-up of urographic abnormalities

If abnormalities are detected on IVU, it may be necessary to proceed to further imaging to obtain additional information and plan further management (Table 3).

> *Key points*
>
> ■ Intravenous urography (IVU) provides both anatomical and functional information, but is appropriate for only a small proportion of urological problems.
>
> ■ A preliminary plain abdominal radiograph is an essential part of the IVU and can often provide a large amount of information.
>
> ■ Intravenous contrast administration is safe, and contrast reactions are unusual, especially with the newer, non-ionic, low-osmolarity agents.
>
> ■ Specific information can be obtained at each stage in the progress of an IVU, and the actual technique may need to be varied according to the findings at each stage.
>
> ■ Some patients require further imaging using other techniques to confirm the diagnosis and plan further management.

Other imaging modalities in urology

Alternatives to conventional radiographs now play a much more significant role in the assessment of urological symptoms. Cross-sectional imaging has become the investigation of choice for staging urological malignancies, and radionuclide studies are widely used for the investigation of kidney function, transplant function and suspected osseous metastases.

Table 1 **Urological indications for cross-sectional imaging**
Renal masses
Staging of urological malignancy
Abscesses, urinomas and infection
Renal/ureteric colic
Renal and lower tract trauma
Retroperitoneum (including adrenal glands)

Cross-sectional imaging

Computerised tomography (CT)
The main indications for CT are shown in Table 1. Thin-slice axial CT avoids superimposition of other structures over the area being studied while individual structures and tissues can be characterised according to their Hounsfield number (Fig. 1). However, axial scanning alone may completely miss or show only part of the lesion (partial volume).

Spiral CT allows images to be obtained over a short period of time (<30 s) and is used to assess suspected

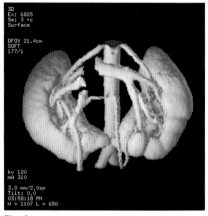

Fig. 2 **Three-dimensional reconstruction of the urinary tract** (CT urogram).

renal colic. Images can be reconstructed in any plane, and three-dimensional (Fig. 2) and vascular reconstruction are also possible; this is useful in the assessment of renal tumours where conservative renal surgery is under consideration. Administration of oral contrast medium outlines bowel, and intravenous contrast allows functional assessment of the kidneys.

Magnetic resonance imaging (MRI)
MRI generates multiplanar images and provides more information than CT about blood flow and static fluid while allowing fat suppression. Tissue characterisation relies on using different pulse sequence parameters (T1 weighting and T2 weighting); T1 weighting is ideal for showing organ anatomy whereas T2 weighting improves visualisation of space-occupying lesions, haematomas and inflammatory processes. Contrast medium (gadolinium) may further improve resolution, and MR angiography produces excellent vascular imaging. The indications for MRI are similar to those for CT, but MRI is

generally better for assessing arterial/venous lesions, lymph nodes and liver parenchyma.

Radionuclide imaging

The radionuclide of choice depends on what function needs to be evaluated.

Renal tubular agents such as ^{99m}Tc-mercaptoacetyltriglycine (MAG3) allow visualisation of the entire urinary tract, especially when renal function is poor, and provide information about vascular uptake by the kidney, distribution within the renal parenchyma and excretion by the kidneys. They are particularly useful for assessing the presence of upper tract obstruction and for investigating renovascular disorders or renal transplant perfusion.

Renal cortical agents such as ^{99m}Tc-dimercaptosuccinic acid (DMSA) are ideal for assessing renal trauma, renal masses, cortical scars and differential function. Such agents give information only about the kidneys and are not useful for assessing ureteric drainage or obstruction.

Bone scintigraphy, using ^{99m}Tc-diphosphonate, is the best means of assessing the presence of osseous metastases in most forms of cancer, but is especially useful in men with carcinoma of the prostate.

Infective foci or abscesses can be assessed using ^{67}gallium citrate or ^{111}indium-labelled white cells.

Adrenal scintigraphy is performed using ^{131}I-iodocholesterol for adrenocortical tumours (Cushing or Conn syndrome) or ^{131}I-meta-iodobenzylguanidine if a medullary tumour (phaeochromocytoma) is suspected.

Direct (using an isotope instilled into the bladder) *or indirect radionuclide cystography* (using MAG3 after it has been excreted into the bladder) is useful for assessing vesicoureteric reflux and with low radiation.

Vascular studies, using ^{99m}Tc-pertechnetate, are helpful in assessing abnormalities of the scrotum (torsion of the testis or epididymitis) when there is concern about impairment of testicular blood flow.

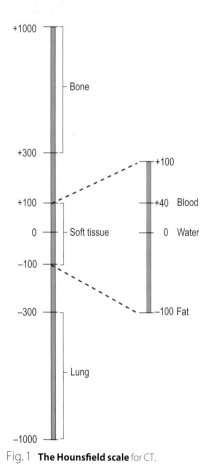

Fig. 1 **The Hounsfield scale** for CT.

Other radiological procedures

Angiography

Cross-sectional imaging has largely replaced angiography in urological assessment. Most angiography is part of an interventional procedure such as angioplasty, thrombolysis, insertion of vascular stents or establishment of vascular access for haemodialysis. Digital subtraction angiography (DSA) is now widely used and produces improved image quality during technically challenging procedures.

Retrograde pyelography

This requires cystoscopy and catheterisation of one or both ureters before the introduction of contrast medium. It is most often used when intravenous urography (IVU) or cross-sectional imaging produces inadequate images of the upper tracts. It may also allow selective urine sampling or brush biopsies for cytological analysis in suspected malignancy, but retrograde ureterorenoscopy is now preferred in these situations.

Cystourethrography

Retrograde cystourethrography is performed by instilling water-soluble contrast medium into the urethra using a small Foley catheter or a special (Knutsson) clamp. It is useful for visualising strictures of the urethra (Fig. 3) and for assessing urethral or bladder trauma. Dynamic studies using radiographic screening during voiding are the best means of assessing the posterior urethra, especially in boys; they may also be used to detect reflux. High pressures should be avoided during contrast instillation, especially when infection is present, and care should be taken in patients with high spinal

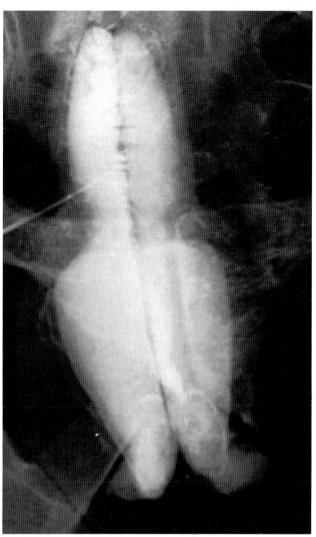

Fig. 4 **Cavernosogram** showing penile 'waisting' due to Peyronie's disease.

cord lesions (above T6) in whom bladder distension may produce life-threatening autonomic dysreflexia.

Cavernosography and vasography

Cavernosography is used occasionally to assess erectile deformity or corporal narrowing produced by Peyronie's disease (Fig. 4). Vasography is now rarely used to assess seminal tract obstruction because sperm aspiration with assisted conception is generally more successful than attempted surgical bypass of obstructive lesions.

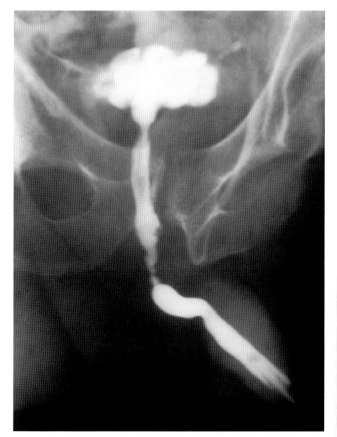

Fig. 3 **Retrograde urethrogram** showing trabeculated bladder and stricture of the bulbar urethra.

> ### Key points
>
> - Cross-sectional imaging using CT or MRI has become the mainstay of urological imaging for renal masses, staging of malignant disease and the investigation of renal colic.
>
> - Spiral CT and rapid acquisition MRI allow multiplanar analysis of images and facilitate two-dimensional or three-dimensional reconstruction as well as allowing indirect angiography.
>
> - Radionuclide imaging is indicated primarily when information is required about kidney function, but is also useful for the assessment of bony metastases and other urological disorders.
>
> - Flexible ureterorenoscopy has largely replaced retrograde pyelography.
>
> - Simple angiography has few diagnostic applications and is usually performed as part of a more complex interventional procedure.

Urodynamic studies

Urodynamic studies produce information on the function of the lower urinary tract (Table 1); when combined with imaging, they are known as videourodynamics. The filling and voiding phases are each studied while the bladder is filled artificially through a catheter. Simple urodynamics only involves measurement of pressure and flow, so limited information can be obtained from such studies (Table 2).

Indications

A urodynamic study may be the key step in patient management (e.g. to confirm bladder outlet obstruction) or simply an additional item of information required to determine overall management. The main indications for urodynamics are shown in Table 3. Urodynamic studies should be performed only to answer specific questions in patients who may wish to proceed with surgical treatment for their symptoms; these studies can be undignified and intimidating so should not be used simply to satisfy the curiosity of the clinician or patient. It should be borne in mind that the filling phase of a urodynamic study (filling cystometry) and pressure flow studies provide data only on pressure, flow and volumes of fluid infused into the bladder and voided, together, occasionally, with images and electromyogram data. Therefore, they can only answer questions using this information. Clinicians sometimes refer patients for urodynamic studies with other questions that cannot be answered by this means, e.g. is there evidence of damage to the cauda equina or does the patient have interstitial cystitis? Questions such as these always require other approaches to answer them, although urodynamic studies may be helpful. In addition, there are intrinsic risks to performing urodynamics, and patients must be made aware of these before agreeing to proceed (Table 4).

Twin-channel urodynamics

This is the usual way in which urodynamic studies are performed. A catheter placed in the bladder measures total bladder pressure. However, this pressure also includes external pressures generated within the abdominal cavity during coughing, straining or movement. A second catheter is therefore placed in the rectum to allow intra-abdominal pressure to be measured. The difference between these two pressures (the subtracted pressure) is a true measure of detrusor pressure.

Urodynamic technique

A twin-lumen catheter (which allows simultaneous filling and pressure recording) or two single-lumen catheters are inserted into the bladder, usually via the urethra; a further catheter is inserted into the rectum to measure intra-abdominal pressure.

In *conventional urodynamics*, the bladder is filled with saline at a rate far greater than would occur during normal bladder filling with urine. If the bladder is filled too quickly, urodynamic abnormalities may be precipitated that have no physiological basis. Filling is usually performed using an external pump with the patient sitting, standing or lying. Continuous recordings are taken of bladder and rectal pressure, together with the subtracted detrusor pressure.

The patient is asked to indicate when filling induces the first sensation of fullness and when the bladder feels

Table 1 **Urodynamic modalities**	
Term	**Information obtained**
Voiding flow rate	Maximum flow during voiding
Residual urine estimate (ultrasound or catheterised)	Urine volume remaining after voiding
Single-channel cystometry	Bladder pressure during filling
Twin-channel subtraction cystometry	Bladder and abdominal pressures during bladder filling and voiding with measurement of flow rate during voiding (pressure flow study)
Videocystometry	Imaging of the urinary tract during urodynamics
Pelvic floor or urethral sphincter electromyography (EMG)	Electrical potentials of periurethral or pelvic floor musculature
Urethral pressure profilometry (UPP)	Pressure along the urethra
Ambulatory cystometry	Bladder and abdominal pressure measurement during normal daily activities or sleep

Table 2 **Conditions that can be assessed by urodynamics**	
During the filling phase	Detrusor overactivity
	Stress urinary incontinence
	Vesicoureteric reflux
	Vesicovaginal and ureterovaginal fistulae
During the voiding phase	Bladder outlet obstruction
	Detrusor hypocontractility
	Detrusor–sphincter dyssynergia

Table 3 **Indications for urodynamics**	
Clinical problem	**Question to be answered**
Symptoms of overactive bladder refractory to conservative measures	Is there detrusor overactivity?
Symptoms of stress incontinence refractory to conservative measures	Is there stress incontinence?
Lower urinary tract symptoms refractory to conservative measures	Is there bladder outlet obstruction?
Chronic retention or voiding symptoms in men before prostatic surgery or in women before surgery for stress incontinence	Is there an underactive (hypocontractile) detrusor?
Voiding symptoms in neurogenic lower urinary tract dysfunction	Is there detrusor–sphincter dyssynergia?
Loin pain in neurogenic lower urinary tract dysfunction	Is there vesicoureteric reflux?
Unexplained post-operative vaginal leakage	Is there a vesicovaginal or ureterovaginal fistula?

Table 4 **Risks of urodynamics**	
Lower urinary tract infection (especially in patients with a history of recurrent urinary infection)	5–10%
Upper urinary tract infection and septicaemia	1%
Acute retention of urine	1–5%
Haematuria	15%

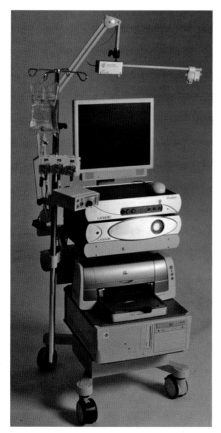

Fig. 1 **The 'stack' of urodynamic equipment.**

'normally' full. Continued filling may then precipitate an urgent need to void. These points are all recorded on the pressure tracing, together with any associated bladder contractions (detrusor overactivity) or episodes of stress incontinence during coughing.

Once the bladder is full, filling is stopped, and the patient is asked to pass urine into a flow rate machine while retaining the pressure-measuring catheters. This allows a measurement of the maximum urinary flow rate and the detrusor pressure that generates voiding. Computer software then determines the presence of obstruction based on nomograms of pressure and flow. In general, low flow with raised detrusor pressure, or normal flow with greatly raised detrusor pressure, are indicative of bladder outlet obstruction.

Urodynamic equipment is available as a 'stack' (Fig. 1), which holds the saline infusion, filling pump, external pressure transducers and the data capture hardware/software.

In *ambulatory urodynamics*, the bladder is allowed to fill naturally with urine over a long period of time, and the pressures may be measured using a recording box that the patient carries around; the recording is later analysed by the urodynamic equipment. It is less commonly used than conventional urodynamics but may be a more accurate reflection of detrusor physiology.

Sphincter electromyography (*EMG*) and *urethral pressure profilometry* (*UPP*) are used only in specialist units for assessment of complex pelvic floor problems.

Videourodynamic studies involve simultaneous fluoroscopic screening of the lower urinary tract with conventional urodynamic measurements. Fluoroscopy may be performed on a tilting table or in a sitting position (which is ideal for women) and images can be stored on computer for later analysis. They are said to be useful when simultaneous evaluation of structure and function is necessary (e.g. bladder neck dysfunction in young men with LUTS, identification of dyssynergia in patients with neuropathic bladders) and when associated pathology such as vesicoureteric reflux is thought to coexist. Many urologists, however, would question the theoretical advantages of videourodynamic studies in patients with uncomplicated lower urinary tract dysfunction.

> ### Key points
>
> ■ A clear understanding of what questions are being asked during a urodynamic study is crucial.
>
> ■ Conventional urodynamics usually implies a simple pressure–flow study.
>
> ■ Because only pressure and flow are recorded, limited conclusions can be drawn from conventional urodynamics.
>
> ■ Urodynamic studies should be performed only when the information obtained may be critical to subsequent patient management.

Infections

Pyelonephritis

Mechanism of infection

Half of patients with acute cystitis also have bacteria in the upper tracts, and the bacteriological pattern of the two conditions is very similar (Table 1). Spread is usually from the faecal reservoir via the urethra, bladder and ureters into the kidney, although some cases are due to haematogenous infection (especially *Staphylococcus aureus* and *Candida* infections). Spread from the bladder does not always require vesicoureteric reflux but is due to fimbriated bacteria, usually *Escherichia coli*, which have the ability to bind to receptors on the epithelial lining. Certain well-defined conditions seem to predispose to the development of pyelonephritis (Table 2). The urinary tract resists the spread of infection by having urine constantly washed through it; Tamm–Horsfall protein (uromucoid) and immunoglobulin A (IgA) in vaginal secretions also play a part in preventing infections.

Acute pyelonephritis

Acute pyelonephritis presents with loin pain, pyrexia and chills. Bacteria, white cells and red cells (in 40–60%) are found in the urine, and there is often tenderness in the loin on examination. The diagnosis of urinary infection is made by the finding of >100 000 organisms/mL on bacterial culture of the urine and/or >10 white cells/mL, but 20% of patients do not have significant bacteriuria. Eighty per cent of infections are due to *E. coli*, and 50% have associated cystitis. A dip slide system can produce more rapid bacteriology results, and the culture process can be initiated immediately. Diabetic patients often have gas-forming organisms in the urine and occasionally develop *emphysematous pyelonephritis* with gas bubbles forming in the renal parenchyma. Patients with upper tract calculi may develop severe *xanthogranulomatous pyelonephritis* with profound bacteraemia and little or no function in the affected kidney.

Imaging techniques are necessary to confirm the diagnosis and to exclude obstruction. An intravenous urogram (IVU) remains the investigation of choice; this may show focal renal enlargement, cortical striations due to oedema and delayed appearance of the nephrogram or pyelogram. The IVU may show gas in the renal parenchyma in diabetic patients. Ultrasound adds little to the diagnostic process, and computerised tomography (CT) is indicated only if the IVU or ultrasound show no abnormality and when xanthogranulomatous pyelonephritis or a renal/perirenal abscess is suspected. Radionuclide studies using ^{99m}Tc-mercaptoacetyltriglycine (MAG3) may help to determine function in the affected kidney, and ^{111}indium-labelled white cells or ^{67}gallium scintigraphy is occasionally used to detect local collections of infection.

Treatment is with a 7-day course of oral antibiotics; a fluoroquinolone (ciprofloxacin, norfloxacin or ofloxacin) is usually preferred. In complicated cases, such as those patients with obstruction or other underlying problems, 14–21 days of treatment may be needed. Xanthogranulomatous pyelonephritis (Fig. 1) usually results in a non-functioning kidney and is best managed by nephrectomy provided the contralateral kidney is functioning normally.

Table 1 **Uropathogenic organisms**	
Ascending infection	**Haematogenous infection**
Bacteria	Bacteria
Escherichia coli	*Mycobacterium tuberculosis*
Klebsiella	*Salmonella typhi*
Proteus	*Staphylococcus aureus*
Pseudomonas	
Streptococcus faecalis	
Staphylococcus saprophyticus	
Staphylococcus epidermidis	
Fungi	Fungi
Candida	*Histoplasma*
	Parasites
	Schistosoma haematobium
	Echinococcus (hydatid disease)
	Viruses
	Cytomegalovirus
	Adenovirus type II
	Human immunodeficiency virus-1

Table 2 **Predispositions to acute pyelonephritis**
Upper tract obstruction of any cause
Calculous hydronephrosis
Urea-splitting organisms (e.g. *Proteus*) because of the stone-forming tendency
Underlying congenital anomalies, especially those causing dilatation or obstruction
Diabetes mellitus
Neuropathic bladder
Indwelling catheter or ureteric stent

Renal and perirenal abscess

Until recently, renal abscesses were mostly caused by haematogenous spread of *S. aureus* or *Candida albicans*, but the pattern has now changed and most are caused by the same organisms that produce acute pyelonephritis. The clinical features are similar to those of acute pyelonephritis but may be more severe, and the abscess usually forms in the renal cortex (Fig. 2). IVU or ultrasound scanning shows a mass in

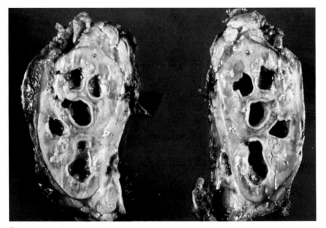

Fig. 1 Nephrectomy specimen showing **xanthogranulomatous pyelonephritis.**

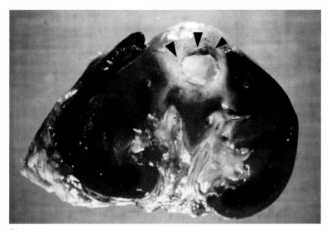

Fig. 2 Nephrectomy specimen showing **a renal cortical abscess** (black arrowheads).

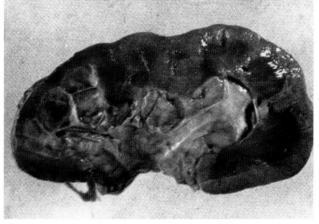

Fig. 3 Post-mortem specimen showing a small, focally scarred kidney resulting from **chronic pyelonephritis.**

the kidney, but CT is the investigation of choice. With small abscesses (<3 cm in diameter), simple antibiotic therapy may be curative, but larger abscesses require drainage by percutaneous puncture or open surgery. Such abscesses may also rupture from the kidney into the perirenal tissue within Gerota's fascia to produce a *perirenal abscess*, for which percutaneous or open surgical drainage is also indicated.

Chronic pyelonephritis

This is defined as a small, scarred kidney (Fig. 3) that may have been affected by previous infection, but it is not always associated with urinary infection. Less than 1% of cases are associated with vesicoureteric reflux (VUR). Chronic pyelonephritis may present with recurrent urinary tract infections but is often detected incidentally. IVU and ultrasound show coarse, focal scarring in the renal cortex, and ^{99m}Tc-dimercaptosuccinic acid (DMSA) scanning shows

cortical defects in the kidney at the site of the scars. A micturating cystogram or an indirect radionuclide cystogram may be useful to demonstrate VUR.

A small proportion of patients with extensive bilateral scarring progress to endstage renal disease and require dialysis or transplantation, but there is no good evidence that chronic pyelonephritis causes hypertension; 7–12% of patients subsequently develop high blood pressure, but this is similar to the risk of hypertension in the normal adult population.

VUR should be treated appropriately, but there is no specific treatment available for chronic pyelonephritis. Patients should be carefully monitored for urinary infection and, if infection or VUR is present, treated with low-dose prophylactic antibiotics; acute infections should be treated vigorously with oral antibiotics. Long-term monitoring is essential to detect progression to chronic renal failure or endstage renal disease.

Key points

- Acute pyelonephritis is caused by the standard uropathogenic bacteria; *E. coli* in 80% of cases.
- Oral antibiotic therapy settles most episodes of acute pyelonephritis, but radiological imaging is essential to exclude predisposing conditions.
- Renal and perirenal abscesses are usually secondary to acute pyelonephritis but may arise as a result of haematogenous spread.
- Chronic pyelonephritis is often asymptomatic and may not require specific treatment unless vesicoureteric reflux is present.
- Chronic pyelonephritis may progress to chronic renal failure and endstage renal disease, but does not cause hypertension in later life.

Lower urinary tract infections

Acute bacterial cystitis

Up to 50% of sexually active women will have at least one attack of cystitis during their lifetime, but infection in men and children is rare. Infection is invariably faecal contamination, via the perineum, with fimbriated bacteria (*Escherichia coli* in 80% of cases). Clinical features include frequency, dysuria, urgency, haematuria and offensive ('fishy') urine. In severe cases, there may be systemic upset with signs of acute pyelonephritis. Abnormal findings on examination are unusual, although there may be suprapubic and pelvic tenderness.

Diagnosis is made by urine culture showing >100 000 organisms/mL and >10 white blood cells/mL. Further investigations in women are unnecessary unless there are signs of upper tract involvement or haematuria persists. In males <50 years, a plain abdominal radiograph (KUB) should be performed to exclude stones, but no other investigations are needed. In older men and children, full assessment of the urinary tract with KUB and ultrasound is necessary.

Treatment is oral antibiotics (a 3-day course on a 'best guess' policy) while awaiting the results of culture and sensitivity; urine culture should be repeated 1 week after treatment to ensure bacterial eradication. The preferred antibiotics are fluoroquinolones (norfloxacin, ciprofloxacin, cephalexin, trimethoprim or ampicillin). In patients >65 years, in patients with diabetes or if symptoms are severe or fail to settle, treatment should be continued for 1 week.

Chronic bacterial cystitis

Chronic bacterial cystitis may be due to re-infection, relapse or persistence of bacteria after previous treatment. Chronic recurrent infection eventually causes squamous metaplasia in the bladder and may progress to squamous carcinoma. Some 95% of cases affect women, and a number of underlying predispositions exist (Table 1). Investigations include urine culture, KUB and ultrasound of the urinary tract; cystoscopy may be necessary in intractable infections to exclude carcinoma of the bladder.

Simple 'self-help' measures (Table 2) are useful, but the mainstay of treatment is low-dose prophylactic antibiotics (trimethoprim, norfloxacin, nitrofurantoin, cephalexin) for 6–12 months; these eliminate recurrence in 95% of patients. In post-menopausal women, estrogen replacement may be necessary, and dilatation of the bladder neck helps some patients with poor bladder emptying.

Table 1 **Predispositions to chronic, recurrent cystitis**
Sexual intercourse (*honeymoon cystitis*)
Post-menopausal estrogen deficiency
Urinary tract calculi
Chronic bacterial prostatitis
Unilateral, infected, atrophic kidney
Foreign bodies in the urinary tract
Intestinovesical fistulae
Diabetes mellitus
Neuropathic bladder

Table 2 **Self-help measures in chronic, recurrent cystitis**
High oral fluid intake (500 mL every 2 h)
Avoid bubble baths, talcum powder and personal deodorants
Oral potassium citrate or sodium bicarbonate
Take proprietary urinary antiseptics
Two-hourly voiding with *double micturition*
Regular washing of introitus using a separate flannel
Wash the perineum from front to back
Lubrication during sexual intercourse (*KY jelly*)
Single antibiotic tablet after sexual intercourse

Abacterial cystitis

Some *Chlamydia*, *Lactobacillus*, *Corynebacteria* and *adenoviral* infections may cause culture-negative cystitis, but often respond to standard antibiotics. *Cyclophosphamide* may produce chronic haemorrhagic cystitis, which may require hydrostatic bladder dilatation, bladder substitution or even urinary diversion. *Radiation cystitis* sometimes follows pelvic irradiation, resulting in bladder contracture and intractable urinary symptoms requiring bladder substitution or urinary diversion. *Interstitial cystitis* is a rare condition of unknown origin characterised by bladder pain, haematuria and lower urinary tract symptoms (see symptom questionnaire, Appendix p. 151). Cystoscopy reveals fissuring of the bladder during filling with bleeding on decompression and occasional ulceration (*Hunner's ulcers*); bladder biopsies show full-thickness inflammation with mast cell infiltration. Treatment can be difficult, but many patients respond to intravesical installations of dimethylsulphoxide (DMSO), oral pentosanpolysulphate or H2-receptor antagonists. Intractable symptoms may respond to hydrostatic bladder dilatation, but may require treatment with oral steroids, bladder substitution or urinary diversion.

| Table 3 **Classification, features and treatment of prostatitis** | | | | |
Type I	Type II	Type IIIa	Type IIIb	Type IV
Acute bacterial	Chronic bacterial	Chronic pelvis pain syndrome (*inflammatory*)	Chronic pelvis pain syndrome (*non-inflammatory*)	Asymptomatic inflammatory (*histological*)
Acute bacterial infection	Recurrent bacterial infection	No demonstrable infection WBCs in prostatic component or voided urine	No WBCs in prostatic component of localisation	No symptoms but found histologically on prostatic biopsy WBCs in EPS and VB3
Fever, low back pain, perineal pain, LUTS or retention of urine	Relapsing urinary infections (usually *E. coli*), suprapubic pain and variable LUTS	Chronic pelvic and perineal pain, irritative LUTS, painful ejaculation, erectile dysfunction, loss of libido	Chronic pelvic and perineal pain, irritative LUTS, worse on sitting and with certain foods, pain before or after ejaculation	Asymptomatic
Pyrexia, tachycardia and exquisite tenderness on rectal examination	Prostate normal, tender, firm or 'boggy'	Prostate normal, tender, firm or 'boggy'	Prostate normal or tender Tender pelvic floor musculature	Prostate normal, tender, firm or 'boggy'
Parenteral antibiotics then oral fluoroquinolone for 4–6 weeks Avoid urethral catheterisation Analgesia and antipyretics	Fluoroquinolone, doxycycline or cephalexin for 6 weeks Alpha-blockers for up to 6 months	Fluroquinolone for 6 weeks Alpha-blockers for up to 6 months; NSAIDs for 6–8 weeks; Regular ejaculation; Repeated prostatic massage; Sitz baths; Transurethral microwave thermotherapy	Fluroquinolone for 6 weeks Alpha-blockers for up to 6 months NSAIDs for 6–8 weeks; Transurethral microwave thermotherapy; Biofeedback and psychological treatment; Local anaesthetic to trigger points	No treatment needed

WBCs, white blood cells; EPS, expressed prostatic secretions; VB3, voided bladder urine.

Asymptomatic bacteriuria

Asymptomatic bacteriuria is seen in 3.5% of the population. In schoolgirls, the incidence is only 1%, but this rises with increasing age at a rate of 1–2% per decade. Women arwnd pregnant women, full investigation and treatment is needed to prevent symptomatic infection. Otherwise, the initial infection is treated with appropriate antibiotics and, provided there is no underlying urological abnormality, no further measures are necessary even if the infection fails to resolve.

Prostatitis

The classification, investigation and management of prostatitis are shown in Table 3; Stamey localisation is the basis for this diagnostic classification (see p. 19). *Acute prostatitis* causes severe symptoms that may require emergency admission; the development of a *prostatic abscess*, seen on computerised tomography (CT) or transrectal ultrasound, is an indication for transurethral drainage.

Epididymitis

Acute epididymitis usually presents with scrotal pain, swelling and reddening; the differential diagnosis includes torsion of the testis and orchitis. Symptoms of urinary infection are present in a minority of patients, but urethral discharge may be seen in younger men.

Diagnosis is made by clinical examination and ultrasound of the scrotum (Fig. 1). In children, the condition is usually due to an underlying urological abnormality, and full investigation with urinary tract ultrasound is required. In men aged <45 years, the spectrum of organisms is similar to that implicated in non-gonococcal urethritis; full genitomedical assessment is needed. In older men, bladder outflow obstruction is the usual cause, and infection results from the usual uropathogenic bacteria.

Treatment is with oral antibiotics (norfloxacin, ciprofloxacin or ofloxacin) and must be continued for at least 6 weeks, although young men respond best to a combination of doxycycline and ofloxacin. A 2-week course of doxycycline is preferred for *Chlamydia*. Involvement of the testis is common (*epididymo-orchitis*), can be detected by ultrasound and may require drainage or orchidectomy if an abscess develops.

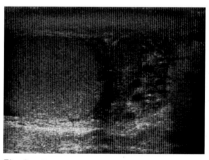

Fig. 1 **Ultrasound of the scrotum in acute epididymitis** showing swollen epididymal tail.

Orchitis

Acute orchitis may complicate any viral illnesses and is particularly common in mumps, rubella or Coxsackie infections. *Mumps orchitis* occurs in 15–20% of affected adults 3–7 days after the parotitis; in 15% of men, the infection is bilateral. The diagnosis is made on the history of parotitis and on detection of circulating antibodies to mumps virus. Analgesia, scrotal support and bedrest are usually effective, but 50% progress to testicular atrophy and, if this is bilateral, infertility may result; steroids are used in bilateral cases to minimise this risk.

> ### Key points
>
> - Acute cystitis is common in women, responds to a short course of antibiotics and only requires detailed investigation in men aged >45 years.
>
> - Chronic cystitis occurs almost exclusively in women and may be precipitated by specific factors; 'self-help' may be effective but, if not, low-dose antibiotic prophylaxis is used.
>
> - Interstitial cystitis is a disabling condition that usually responds to intravesical instillations but may require steroids or surgical intervention.
>
> - Prostatitis is a major cause of pelvic pain in men and is difficult to treat effectively.
>
> - Epididymitis requires prolonged treatment with antibiotics to prevent chronicity.

Human immunodeficiency virus and the urinary tract

In 1981, health monitoring authorities in the USA detected a dramatic rise in the incidence of pneumocystic pneumonia, Kaposi's sarcoma and other opportunistic infections in the homosexual community of Los Angeles and New York; this marked the start of the acquired immunodeficiency syndrome (AIDS) epidemic.

Table 1 **Modes of spread of HIV-1**	
Sexual transmission	Male homosexuals or bisexuals in the developed world
	Heterosexuals in developing countries
Blood or blood products	Intravenous drug users
	Haemophiliacs (contaminated factor VIII)
Vertical transmission	Transplacental
	During birth (by blood droplets)
	In breast milk

Epidemiology

The human immunodeficiency virus (HIV-1) probably arose in the African subcontinent by mutation of a primate strain (HIV-2), and was then propagated by heterosexual transmission. The commonest modes of spread are shown Table 1. There is good evidence from African studies that circumcision protects against the heterosexual transmission of HIV-1 by removing the virus-laden inner layer of the prepuce.

Virology

HIV-1 is a *retrovirus* belonging to the *lentivirus* family. It is an enveloped RNA virus with a 9200-nucleotide genome. It binds to CD4 receptors on the surface of helper T-lymphocytes (CD4+ T cells) and penetrates into the cell, where it sheds its outer envelope. Reverse transcriptase then produces a DNA provirus that integrates into the cell genome, resulting in synthesis and maturation of virus progeny (Fig. 1). The virus

does not result in cell lysis, so infection tends to be permanent. It normally affects macrophage cells and, as a result, localises in regional lymph nodes; as these macrophages are killed off by the virus, immunodeficiency results.

Clinical features

The main clinical features of HIV-1 infection are shown in Table 2.

Urological manifestations

Involvement of the genitourinary tract is usually by opportunistic infection due to immunosuppression or by the development of malignancy, although there are also some urological disorders that are specific to HIV-1 infection.

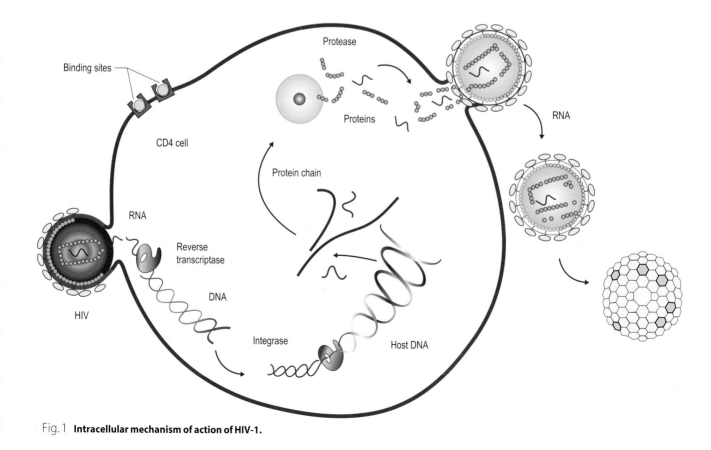

Fig. 1 **Intracellular mechanism of action of HIV-1.**

Table 2 **Clinical patterns associated with HIV-1 infection**

1. Seroconversion illness	Seen in 10% within a few weeks of exposure
	Coincides with seroconversion
	Glandular fever-like illness
2. Incubation period	8–10 years (usually asymptomatic)
3. AIDS-related complex or persistent generalised lymphadenopathy (PGL)	
4. Full-blown AIDS	
5. Other manifestations	Encephalopathy (in 65%)
	Skin eruptions
	Persistent diarrhoea

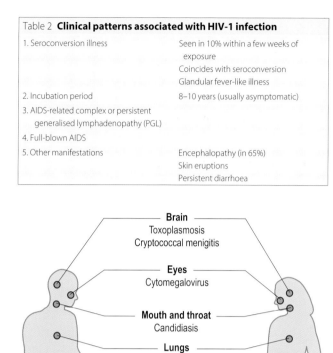

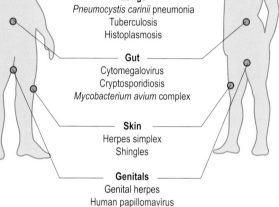

Fig. 2 **Opportunistic infections in HIV-1 infection.**

Brain
Toxoplasmosis
Cryptococcal menigitis

Eyes
Cytomegalovirus

Mouth and throat
Candidiasis

Lungs
Pneumocystis carinii pneumonia
Tuberculosis
Histoplasmosis

Gut
Cytomegalovirus
Cryptosporidiosis
Mycobacterium avium complex

Skin
Herpes simplex
Shingles

Genitals
Genital herpes
Human papillomavirus
Vaginal candidiasis

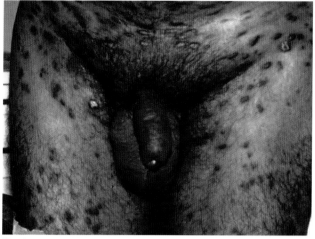

Fig. 3 **Genital lesions in Kaposi's sarcoma.**

Table 3 **Antiretroviral agents**

Nucleoside analogue reverse transcriptase inhibitors, e.g. azidothymidine, lamivudine
Non-nucleotide analogue reverse transcriptase inhibitors, e.g. nevirapine
Protease inhibitors, e.g. indinavir, ritonavir

Opportunistic infection (Fig. 2)

Infections of the kidneys can occur with *cytomegalovirus, Aspergillus* or *Toxoplasma gondii. Cytomegalovirus* is often associated with acute tubular necrosis and with widespread disease. Aspergillosis and toxoplasmosis usually respond to systemic treatment, but may cause abscesses that require drainage or nephrectomy. *Herpes simplex virus infections* and *venereal warts* are often recurrent, and transmission to sexual partners is a major risk. Syphilis and Reiter's disease may also occur, often in atypical forms. In women, *pelvic inflammatory disease* may be severe enough to require surgical intervention. Up to 25% of patients may have a superimposed *urinary infection,* and bacterial prostatitis may also occur. *Infection in the testis or epididymis* is seen in up to 40% of patients at autopsy and, if symptomatic, may be prolonged or fulminant with abscess formation.

Urological malignancies

A wide range of malignancies has been reported, including squamous cell carcinoma, malignant melanoma, testicular cancer and lymphoreticular neoplasms. Women are particularly at risk of cervical carcinoma, and regular cervical screening is recommended for infected women. Kaposi's sarcoma in the genital region (Fig. 3) is seen in up to 20% of HIV-positive patients.

Other urological disease

HIV nephropathy is seen in 5–10% of infected patients and is characterised by proteinuria, uraemia and focal segmental glomerulosclerosis on renal biopsy. Progression to renal failure is uncommon but, if peritoneal dialysis is required, the prognosis is poor (2-year survival rate of 50%). Upper tract calculi can arise in patients treated with indinavir because of crystallisation of the drug within the urinary tract; stones may be dissolved by stopping the drug temporarily and by urinary acidification (pH < 4). Urinary retention, lower urinary tract symptoms and detrusor hyper-reflexia are seen in 25–50% of patients and are best managed in the standard manner. Microscopic haematuria is seen in 25% of affected patients and does not require full urological evaluation.

Management

Vaccines against HIV-1 have proved difficult to develop because of the variability of different HIV-1 strains (due to alterations in the viral envelope) and because animal models are unreliable. However, a number of drugs are available for the treatment of HIV-1 infection (Table 3). The usual treatment strategy is to employ two nucleoside analogue reverse transcriptase inhibitors in combination with a protease inhibitor; this minimises drug resistance and may ultimately reduce toxicity.

> *Key points*
>
> ■ HIV-1 infection has become a major health problem since 1981, although changes in the sexual practices of homosexuals in particular have limited the spread of the disease.
>
> ■ Urological manifestations are related to opportunistic infections, development of malignancy and specific genitourinary problems.
>
> ■ Treatment using multiple drug regimes is highly effective.
>
> ■ Prevention is better than cure.

Urinary tract infection in childhood

Background

Two per cent of boys and 8% of girls will have a urinary tract infection (UTI) during their childhood. In boys, 80% of infections happen during the first year of life, probably due to subpreputial organisms. In the absence of a congenital anomaly, the longer male urethra affords protection until school age. In girls, the peak incidence is at school age.

Investigation is vital and shows a urinary tract anomaly in up to 40% of cases (Table 1). Renal scarring is usually associated with vesicoureteric reflux (VUR).

Diagnosis

Infants may present with non-specific symptoms (fever, vomiting, diarrhoea and, occasionally, febrile convulsions), chronic ill health or failure to thrive. Boys occasionally present with epididymo-orchitis. Older children have a more organ-specific presentation related to the site of infection. There may be significant morbidity associated with childhood UTI; septicaemia and even death may follow in untreated patients, while scarring of the kidneys may lead to hypertension and renal failure. Urine culture should be performed before starting antibiotic therapy whenever non-specific symptoms suggest UTI.

In infants, a self-adhesive collecting bag is attached to the perineum to collect urine; a catheter or suprapubic needle aspiration may also be used. Older children can provide a midstream or clean catch urine specimen. Cultured organisms are routinely tested against common antibiotics, but treatment may be started before the results are available on a 'best guess' basis.

Management

Antibiotics are usually given orally, with paracetamol or a non-steroidal anti-inflammatory drug to control fever. Intravenous antibiotics and fluid replacement are indicated in children unable to tolerate oral drugs or for organisms resistant to oral antibiotics; this usually requires hospitalisation. Urinary drainage with a urethral catheter may hasten recovery if the bladder is failing to empty.

Table 1 The incidence of urinary tract anomalies found on investigation of UTI in children	
Vesicoureteric reflux (with scarring in 14.5%)	29%
Dilated ureter (PUJ or VUJ)	4.5%
Duplication of the ureter	4.5%
Other anomalies	2%

PUJ, pelviureteric junction; VUJ, vesicoureteric junction.

Table 2 Indications for specific investigations	
Investigation	**Application**
Ultrasound	All patients
^{99m}Tc-dimercaptosuccinic acid (DMSA) scan	Patients less than 1 year old and/or severe UTI (hospitalised)
Micturating cysto-urethrogram (MCUG)	Patients less than 1 year old + dilatation on ultrasound or abnormal DMSA
MAG3 indirect cystogram	Older child (> 3 years) instead of MCUG

Other investigations

Until an underlying congenital urinary anomaly has been excluded, prophylactic antibiotics (usually trimethoprim at 2 mg/kg given once at night) should be given.

The available investigations and their indications are listed in Table 2. ^{99m}Tc-dimercaptosuccinic acid (DMSA) scintigraphy requires an intravenous injection of radionuclide, but is the most sensitive means of detecting renal parenchymal damage (Fig. 1). Micturating cysto-urethrogram (MCUG) requires a catheter, which can be distressing for an older child, but is used to demonstrate reflux in infants and to exclude urethral valves in boys (Fig. 2). ^{99m}Tc-mercaptoacetyltriglycine (MAG3) indirect cystography (Fig. 3) demonstrates reflux without the need for catheterisation.

If an underlying anomaly is found, treatment can be appropriately

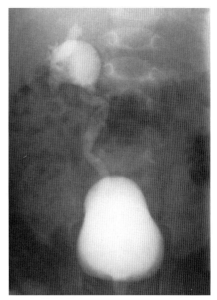

Fig. 2 Micturating cysto-urethrogram (MCUG) showing **grade 3 reflux into the right kidney.** The bladder and urethra are normal.

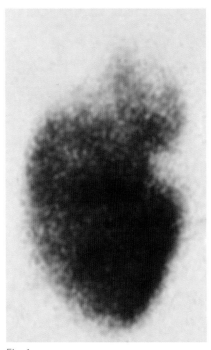

Fig. 1 ^{99m}Tc-dimercaptosuccinic acid (DMSA) scan showing the characteristic **polar scarring of pyelonephritis.**

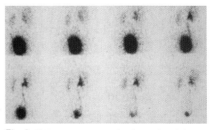

Fig. 3 ^{99m}Tc-mercaptoacetyltriglycine (MAG3) **indirect cystography.** From top left to bottom right, there is evidence of isotope reflux into the right renal pelvis on voiding and a small residue of urine in the bladder at the end.

directed. This usually involves prophylactic antibiotics to see whether further infection can be prevented. Risk factors for recurrent infection are bladder dysfunction, constipation, obstruction or dilatation in the urinary tract, stones and VUR. Additional measures to prevent recurrence include probiotics (bio-yogurt and/or lactobacilli) and vitamin C with treatment of any bladder dysfunction or constipation.

Vesicoureteric reflux

Vesicoureteric reflux is seen in 0.4–1.8% of the paediatric population but in 20–50% of children with a UTI; it is the likely cause of pyelonephritic scarring of the kidney. Organisms pass up the ureter from the bladder into the collecting ducts and cause renal parenchymal damage; this is typically at the upper or lower poles into compound renal papillae. Refluxed urine returning to the bladder after voiding may make it difficult for children with reflux to eliminate infection.

Reflux may be primary (due to a defective valvular mechanism at the vesicoureteric junction) or secondary to increased bladder pressure; the latter is seen in neuropathic bladder and posterior urethral valves. With primary reflux, maturation of the valvular mechanism with time may lead to spontaneous resolution, so treatment is expectant with prophylactic antibiotics.

The diagnosis of reflux is made by MCUG, and the severity is graded according to the degree of dilatation of the ureter and renal collecting system (Table 3). Minor forms of reflux (grades 1 or 2) rarely cause renal damage and have a high spontaneous resolution rate during the early years of life; dilating reflux (grades 3–5) carries a higher risk of renal damage and less chance of spontaneous resolution.

Indications for surgical intervention include recurrent infections, progressive renal damage and non-compliance with medical management. Reflux is now usually corrected by injecting an inert paste cystoscopically under the ureteric orifice to change its shape and recreate the valvular mechanism. Open reimplantation of the ureter is reserved for patients with high-grade reflux whose large ureteric orifices are not amenable to injections.

Many patients with reflux are identified following antenatal diagnosis of a dilated kidney. Treatment of these patients is expectant and follows the guidelines above. Some already have an abnormal kidney at birth without ever having had a UTI, and reflux may simply be one manifestation of general maldevelopment or dysplasia of the kidney.

Table 3 **International classification of the severity of vesicoureteric reflux**

Grade	Description	Spontaneous resolution rate
1	Into a non-dilated ureter	83%
2	Into the pelvis and calyces without dilatation	60%
3	Mild to moderate dilatation of the ureter, renal pelvis and calyces with minimal forniceal blunting	46%
4	Moderate ureteric tortuosity and dilatation of the pelvis and calyces	9%
5	Gross dilatation of the ureter, pelvis and calyces with loss of papillary impressions and ureteric tortuosity	0%

Key points

- UTI occurs in 2% of boys and 8% of girls during childhood and is often associated with congenital anomalies of the urinary tract.
- Diagnosis requires a high index of suspicion, particularly in infants.
- Confirmation with a formal urinary culture is essential, although antibiotics may be started before the results are available.
- All children require investigation with at least an ultrasound scan of their urinary tract.
- The commonest underlying problem is vesicoureteric reflux, and this is likely to be the mechanism of renal damage.
- Treatment of reflux is with prophylactic antibiotics, and there is a high rate of spontaneous resolution.

Assessment of patients with stone disease

Initial patient assessment must be regarded as only part of an ongoing process intended to establish the diagnosis, control symptoms, render the patient stone free and prevent stone recurrence.

History

Colicky loin pain, radiating to the groin and scrotum (in men) or the labia (in women), is typical; constipation and abdominal distension may also be present due to a secondary paralytic ileus. Dysuria, frequency, urgency and strangury may occur with calculi in the intramural ureter. A family history is important, together with a history of previous stones, and details should be sought of drug consumption, prolonged periods of dehydration or visits to hot, dry climates.

Examination

There are often few physical signs, but there may be tenderness in the loin and over the site of the stone. The patient is often restless with tachycardia or hypertension, and may be pyrexial if there is superimposed urinary infection.

Laboratory tests

Urine testing reveals blood in >90% of stone patients; sterile pyuria, crystalluria (cystine, urate and struvite) and evidence of urinary infection may also be seen. Bacteriological examination of the urine should be performed to exclude infection. Measurement of early-morning urinary pH may also be helpful in preventing further stone formation. All patients should be screened for cystinuria using a simple stick test.

Blood tests should include full blood count, renal function (including creatinine and bicarbonate), bone function and uric acid; parathyroid hormone levels should be measured if the corrected serum calcium is raised.

Metabolic screening

The investigations above are sufficient assessment in most patients. In patients less than 30 years old, those with a strong family history of stones, those with recurrent stones (within 5 years) and those with multiple stones, more detailed metabolic assessment is necessary (Table 1).

Imaging

Ninety per cent of calculi will be visible on a *plain abdominal radiograph* due to the presence of calcium or sulphur in the stone.

The most sensitive, definitive investigation is *helical computerised tomography* (CT); *intravenous urography* (IVU) is used if CT is not available.

Ultrasound has a poor detection rate for ureteric calculi and should be used only if CT is not available or if the patient is allergic to contrast medium (Table 2); it is best reserved for lower tract calculi and assessment of bladder outflow obstruction.

Retrograde ureterography or *ureterorenoscopy* may be needed if uncertainty remains about the presence of a stone. CT should not be used during pregnancy; pregnant women with suspected renal colic should be investigated with ultrasound (during the first trimester) or by IVU (in the second and third trimesters).

Radionuclide renography may be helpful in certain situations. ^{99m}Tc-dimercaptosuccinic acid (DMSA) scintigraphy is used to assess relative renal function in patients with staghorn calculi, and ^{99m}Tc-mercaptoacetyltriglycine (MAG3) scintigraphy helps to assess the need for intervention by measuring ureteric obstruction and its effect on renal function.

Stone analysis

Chemical stone analysis may be useful in first-time stone formers, but simple analysis may not accurately reflect stone composition. More detailed stone analysis is indicated for complex stones (Table 1), but the widespread use of lithotripsy means that few intact calculi are presented for analysis. Chemical analysis also helps to rule out 'factitious' calculi. Scanning electron microscopy (Fig. 1) or polarising microscopy may demonstrate crystal structure, but are not routinely used. Stone analysis is particularly useful to detect unusual stone components such as cystine or to detect the presence of foreign bodies within the stone (Fig. 2).

Indications for surgical intervention

Intervention for renal calculi is usually synonymous with stone elimination, but alternative methods may be used for ureteric calculi. In acute ureteric colic, *percutaneous nephrostomy* or *retrograde ureteric stenting* are often used to relieve ureteric obstruction, severe symptoms and infection proximal to a calculus. The indications for surgical intervention are shown in Table 3.

Factors determining treatment options

Many factors determine the choice of treatment for an individual stone (Table 4). Treatment decisions must be tailored to the specific needs of the patient, the stone(s) and the clinical condition as well as the availability of the various treatment modalities.

Table 1 **Full metabolic screening for complex stones**
24-h urine collection (in acid container) for calcium, phosphate, oxalate and citrate
24-h urine collection (without acid) for urate, sodium and creatinine
24-h urine volume measurement (to ensure adequate fluid intake) performed as part of the above
Detailed stone analysis (infrared spectroscopy, X-ray diffraction, optical crystallography)

Table 2 Accuracy of imaging modalities for ureteric calculi

Imaging technique	Positive predictive value	Negative predictive value	Accuracy
Helical CT	97%	100%	98%
Plain radiograph	90%	51%	70%
IVU	93%	31%	60%
Ultrasound	100%	30%	46%

CT, computerised tomography; IVU, intravenous urogram.

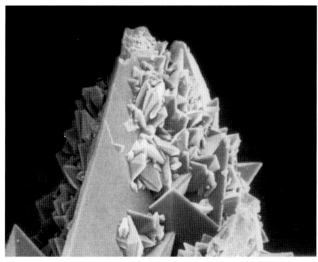

Fig. 1 Scanning electron micrograph showing crystalline structure of a **pure calcium oxalate calculus.**

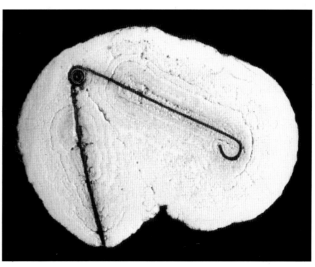

Fig. 2 **Bladder stone** containing a hair grip at its centre.

Table 3 **Indications for surgical intervention**

Failure of conservative measures to relieve symptoms

Ureteric calculi > 7 mm in presenting diameter

Ureteric calculi between 5 and 7 mm that have failed to pass after a trial of conservative management

Impairment of renal function due to obstruction

Proximal infection due to stone impaction and obstruction

Structural abnormalities predisposing to stone formation that require correction to prevent stone recurrence

Table 4 **Factors determining treatment options**

Patient related	Stone related	Clinical factors
Obesity (renders lithotripsy less effective)	Stone burden (lithotripsy retreatment more likely for larger calculi)	General health (fitness for general anaesthesia)
Body habitus (may inhibit imaging during lithotripsy)	Stone composition (oxalate and cystine stones respond poorly to lithotripsy)	Anticoagulation (must be stopped before invasive procedures or lithotripsy)
Pregnancy (lithotripsy is contraindicated)	Stone morphology (smooth-surfaced stones respond less well to lithotripsy)	Aspirin, dipyridamole, clopidogrel (increase the risk of bleeding after intervention)
Renal anatomy (poor stone elimination from calyces that have narrow necks, are dependent or lie at an acute angle to the ureter)	Impacted ureteric calculi (poor fragment elimination)	Urinary infection (treatment may result in bacteraemia)
Symptoms (only 30% of asymptomatic stones progress to symptomatic)		

Key points

■ Calcium oxalate ± phosphate is the commonest type of urinary stone.

■ Low urine volume is the single commonest abnormality predisposing to stone formation and can easily be reversed to minimise stone recurrence.

■ Helical (spiral) CT is the investigation of choice for assessing patients with suspected upper tract calculi.

■ Metabolic abnormalities must be identified and corrected but, despite prevention, the risk of stone recurrence is 50% within 5–7 years with an annual recurrence rate of 7%.

■ Treatment of individual stones must take into account factors related to the patient and his/her general clinical condition as well as the stone itself.

Renal calculi

Treatment options

Symptomatic renal calculi usually require treatment. Symptoms result from movement within the collecting system, superimposed infection or impaction at anatomical narrowings such as calyceal necks, calyceal diverticula or the pelviureteric junction. Small, asymptomatic, calyceal calculi require no treatment, but should be kept under observation by regular plain radiograph, especially if multiple. Enlargement, infection or the subsequent development of symptoms (seen in 30%) should prompt surgical intervention. The common sites for renal calculi are shown in Fig. 1.

The aim of treatment is to produce maximal clearance of stones with minimal morbidity. The available treatment options are shown in Table 1.

Extracorporeal shockwave lithotripsy (ESWL)

Some 80–85% of renal calculi are suitable for ESWL using a lithotriptor (Fig. 2). This generates shock waves within a water cushion by repetitive discharges; these shock waves are focused on the calculus using a hemiellipsoid reflector. The patient lies on the water cushion, and the shock waves pass through the skin to impact with the calculus; accurate targeting is providing by real-time ultrasound scanning or fluoroscopy. Each shock wave produces minor stone fragmentation, and up to 3500 shocks are needed to disintegrate a calculus. Patients may require sedoanalgesia, and antibiotics are given routinely to prevent bacteraemia, but ESWL can usually be accomplished on a daycase basis. The stone fragments are then passed spontaneously over the next 3–4 months.

Calculi larger than 2 cm in diameter run the risk of ureteric obstruction by stone fragments (*steinstrasse*) in up to 10% of cases, although this can be prevented by inserting a ureteric stent prior to ESWL; percutaneous nephrolithotomy (PCNL) may be preferable for larger calculi. Poor response to ESWL is seen in dependent calyceal calculi, obese patients, calculi in diverticula, cystine calculi and pure calcium oxalate calculi; in these patients, PCNL is often preferred. Staghorn calculi (Fig. 3) respond poorly to ESWL monotherapy with low (<50%) stone-free rates; PCNL is preferred with ESWL for any fragments remaining after surgery (85% stone-free rate).

Retreatment is needed for 20% of stones <1 cm and more often for larger stones (up to 45% for stones >2 cm). Haematuria (lasting 12–24 h), ureteric colic (in up to 20%), skin damage (due to shock wave entry and exit), pancreatitis and lung damage are all seen after ESWL. In the long term, there may be permanent functional impairment, an increased risk of stone recurrence and hypertension due to ESWL-induced microvascular damage.

Percutaneous nephrolithotomy (PCNL)

PCNL is the treatment of choice for staghorn calculi and for larger (>2 cm) calculi unresponsive to ESWL or retrograde ureterorenoscopy (URS); it is the best option for calculi in a calyceal diverticulum. The collecting system is opacified with contrast medium and punctured percutaneously. A guidewire is then screened into the kidney and a track dilated into the collecting system to allow the introduction of a rigid nephroscope. Large calculi are broken using laser, ballistic, electrohydraulic or ultrasonic lithotripsy, and all small fragments are extracted. A nephrostomy tube is inserted for

Table 1	**Treatment options for renal calculi**
Minimally invasive	Extracorporeal shock wave lithotripsy (ESWL)
	Percutaneous nephrolithotomy (PCNL)
	Retrograde ureterorenoscopy (URS)
	Laparoscopic stone removal
Open surgery	Pyelolithotomy (for stones in the renal pelvis)
	Nephrolithotomy (for stones in renal calyces)
	Pyelonephrolithotomy (for staghorn calculi)
	Nephrectomy
Stone dissolution	Irrigation with saline, heparin or citrate solutions
Medical treatment	Non-specific: advice about diet and fluid intake
	Specific: treatment of metabolic abnormalities

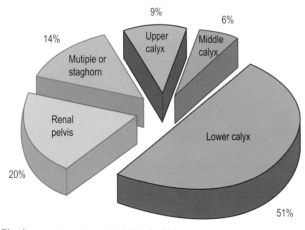

Fig. 1 **The sites of calculi within the kidney.**

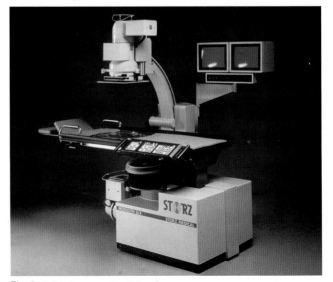

Fig. 2 **A third-generation lithotriptor.**

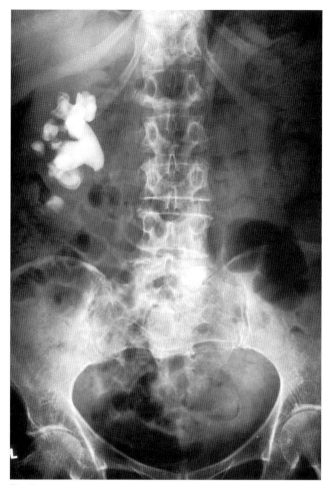

Fig. 3 Plain abdominal radiograph showing a **staghorn calculus** in the right kidney.

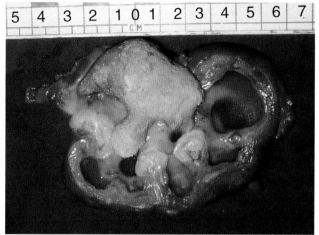

Fig. 4 Nephrectomy specimen showing a **staghorn calculus in a non-functioning, infected, hydronephrotic kidney.**

function (less than 10% of overall function) are best managed by open nephrectomy (Fig. 4). *Xanthogranulomatous pyelonephritis*, where the kidney is destroyed by a combination of stones and locally infiltrative perinephric infection, usually requires open nephrectomy.

Stone dissolution

Stone dissolution is reserved for those patients with multiple residual calculi after ESWL or PCNL in whom further intervention is unlikely to be effective. Irrigation with saline, heparin or citrate solution via a nephrostomy tube or ureteric catheter may, over a period of days, result in stone dissolution. Any urinary infection must be treated vigorously before irrigation is commenced.

Medical treatment (see p. 61)

24–48 h post-operatively. Any residual calculi can be treated by repeat PCNL, irrigation or ESWL.

Retrograde ureterorenoscopy (URS)

The role of URS for renal calculi is limited to calculi <3 cm in diameter in a calyx or a calyceal diverticulum, when ESWL has failed or the calculi are inaccessible to PCNL; it is also used in obese patients where ESWL or PCNL are unlikely to succeed. Using a flexible ureteroscope under fluoroscopic screening, intrarenal calculi can be dislodged into the renal pelvis or upper calyx using stone baskets and disintegrated using holmium laser lithotripsy.

Laparoscopic stone removal

Laparoscopic stone removal is rarely indicated for renal calculi, but may be used to extract calculi from the kidney during laparoscopic pyeloplasty.

Open stone surgery

Minimally invasive methods are generally preferred to open surgery for renal calculi. Staghorn calculi with very poor renal

Key points

- ESWL is the treatment of choice for 80–85% of renal calculi.
- PCNL is used for staghorn calculi and for larger stones (> 2 cm) that are not amenable to ESWL.
- Open surgery is indicated primarily to perform nephrectomy for a non-functioning kidney containing stones.
- Medical treatment may allow dissolution of a small proportion of calculi, but is primarily an adjunct to surgical management in preventing stone recurrence.

Ureteric calculi

Treatment options

Ureteric calculi usually pass spontaneously without the need for surgical intervention. This is related primarily to stone size. The spontaneous passage rates for calculi <4 mm, 4–6 mm and >6 mm are 80%, 60% and 20% respectively. Calculi in the upper ureter are least likely to pass spontaneously (45%), whereas 70% of distal calculi pass. If a ureteric calculus impacts, it usually does so at the pelviureteric junction, the pelvic brim or the ureterovesical junction.

Obstruction and loss of function also determine the need for intervention. Function is rarely lost within the first 2 weeks but may become total after 6 weeks; recovery after relief of obstruction may take up to 3 months. One-third of kidneys obstructed for more than 4 weeks undergo irreversible renal damage, regardless of stone size. Spontaneous passage of a calculus may be encouraged by insertion of a percutaneous nephrostomy, which relieves obstruction, drains infection and restores coaptive peristalsis in the ureter.

Treatment options include extracorporeal shock wave lithotripsy (ESWL), ureteroscopy, open surgery and laparoscopic surgery; percutaneous nephrolithotomy (PCNL) is only appropriate for stones in the upper ureter. In practice, management depends on whether the calculus lies above or below the pelvic brim.

Calculi above the pelvic brim (30%)

ESWL is the treatment of choice for stones in the proximal ureter, with rigid ureteroscopy reserved for failure of fragmentation; the best results are obtained with stones <1 cm in diameter. ESWL can be performed in situ, or the stone can be dislodged back into the kidney by retrograde flushing (*push–bang technique*). Routine use of ureteric stents prior to ESWL is no longer recommended for upper ureteric calculi because of failure to improve fragmentation rates and the risk of encrustation (Fig. 1). The stone-free rates after these interventions are shown in Table 1, but impacted calculi are relatively resistant to ESWL.

The results of ureteroscopy have been dramatically improved by the use of flexible ureteroscopes and laser lithotripsy, which give 95% stone-free rates with minimal morbidity. Flexible ureteroscopy with laser lithotripsy is the treatment of choice for cystine calculi, impacted stones, obese patients, patients with coagulation disorders and calculi >1 cm. The stone fragments are usually left in situ to pass alongside a ureteric stent inserted for 2–4 weeks. If ureteroscopic disintegration fails, PCNL may be considered, either by direct removal of the calculus from the proximal ureter or following its dislodgement back into the kidney (*push–pull technique*).

Laparoscopic stone removal and open surgery are indicated only as 'salvage' procedures when all other methods have failed.

Calculi below the pelvic brim (70%)

The stone-free rates for distal ureteric calculi are shown in Table 2; there is little to choose between ESWL and rigid ureteroscopy for distal ureteric calculi. At ureteroscopy (Fig. 2), calculi <4 mm may be extracted without disintegration using a stone basket (Fig. 3) or grasping forceps; calculi >4 mm usually require disintegration using ballistic, electrohydraulic, ultrasonic or laser lithotripsy followed by fragment extraction. A ureteric stent is usually left in situ after ureteroscopy if calculi >2 mm remain after fragmentation or if there has been evidence of ureteric trauma during the procedure.

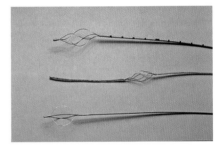

Fig. 2 Different types of **stone retrieval baskets.**

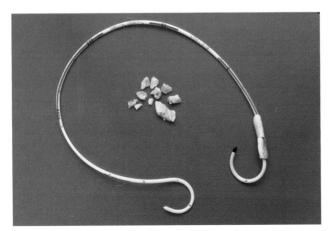

Fig. 1 **Encrusted ureteric stent** left in situ for 6 months during ESWL to a proximal ureteric calculus.

Table 1 **Stone-free rates for interventions on ureteric calculi above the pelvic brim**

Stone size	Modality	Stone-free rate
<1 cm	ESWL	84%
	Ureteroscopy	56%
>1 cm	ESWL	72%
	Ureteroscopy	44%

Table 2 **Stone-free rates for interventions on ureteric calculi below the pelvic brim**

Stone size	Modality	Stone-free rate
<1 cm	ESWL	85%
	Ureteroscopy	89%
>1 cm	ESWL	74%
	Ureteroscopy	73%

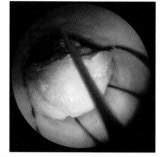

Fig. 3 **Ureteroscopic basket extraction** of a ureteric calculus.

Table 3 **Patient advice on diet and fluid intake to prevent recurrent stones**

Constituent	Advice
Fluid	Increase fluid intake to maintain colourless urine (3 L/24 h)
Protein	Decrease intake below 52 g/24 h to limit urate excretion, calcium excretion and oxalate supersaturation
Salt	Restrict intake to below 50 mmol/24 h to lower urinary calcium excretion
Oxalate	Reduce oxalate intake from strawberries, rhubarb, spinach, chocolate and nuts Avoid vitamin C supplements, which increase oxalate excretion
Calcium	Maintain normal calcium intake above 30 mmol/24 h (low-calcium diets cause increased urinary oxalate levels)
Dietary fibre	Increase intake of fibre to reduce calcium absorption from the gut
Cranberry juice	Daily cranberry juice decreases urinary oxalate and phosphate and increases urinary citrate

The use of flexible ureteroscopes and laser lithotripsy has reduced the complication rate of ureteroscopy to <1%; perforation, strictures, ureteric avulsion and loss of the calculus outside the ureter may all occur.

PCNL is not indicated for distal ureteric calculi. Laparoscopic surgery (transperitoneal or retroperitoneal) may be used for calculi unresponsive to ESWL and inaccessible to ureteroscopy. Open surgery is indicated only as a 'salvage' procedure when all else has failed.

Ureteric steinstrasse

Following ESWL to renal calculi >2 cm in diameter, multiple fragments may obstruct the ureter (*steinstrasse*); 70% occur in the lower ureter. The risk of this may be prevented by prophylactic ureteric stenting before ESWL. Some 80–90% resolve spontaneously, and this may be assisted by percutaneous nephrostomy tube insertion. A steinstrasse that fails to resolve after 3–4 weeks is best treated by ureteroscopic extraction or by ESWL to the leading stone fragment.

Medical treatment

Non-specific advice about diet and fluid intake (Table 3) should be given to all stone patients and reduces recurrent stones by up to 85% in patients who do not have hypercalciuria.

Specific medical therapy for stones is used as an adjunct to surgery and to prevent further stone formation. *Thiazide diuretics* reduce the risk of recurrent stones in patients with hypercalciuria by reducing urinary calcium excretion. Protein restriction, *allopurinol* and urinary alkalinisation (to keep the urinary pH between 6.2 and 6.5) help to reduce hyperuricosuria. Enteric hyperoxaluria usually responds to oxalate restriction or, if this fails, to oral pyridoxine (100 mg daily). Hypocitraturia is managed by oral potassium or sodium citrate supplements. Cystine stones can occasionally be dissolved by increasing urine output to 3 L/24 h and by alkalinising the urine (pH >7.5); chelating agents such as *D-penicillamine* or *α-mercaptopropionylglycine* (MCG) are also used, but side-effects (e.g. nephrotoxicity) limit their use. Urease inhibitors are no longer used for struvite (infective) stones because of their toxicity.

Bladder, urethral and other calculi

Bladder calculi make up approximately 5% of all urinary calculi and urethral calculi <1%.

Bladder calculi

In underdeveloped countries, bladder calculi are common in children, are caused by a poor diet combined with chronic dehydration and are usually composed of ammonium urate (Fig. 1). In developed countries, bladder calculi are usually struvite (infective); occasionally, they are composed of calcium oxalate and take on the appearance of 'jackstones' (Fig. 2).

Clinical features

Presentation is usually in men over the age of 50 years, and there are frequently associated symptoms of bladder outflow obstruction. Calculi may also develop in neurogenic bladders, on foreign bodies in the bladder and within bladder diverticula. Calculi that pass down from the upper tracts very rarely remain and enlarge in the bladder.

The presence of obstructive or irritative lower urinary tract symptoms (LUTS) and dysuria, haematuria, suprapubic pain or sudden interruption of the urinary stream should suggest the presence of a bladder calculus. Specific findings on examination are unusual.

Investigations

Metabolic investigations are not usually necessary, but a midstream urine should be checked for infection. Diagnosis is by plain abdominal radiograph (Fig. 3), abdominal ultrasound or computerised tomography (CT). Cystoscopy and specific assessment of LUTS may also be needed for a full assessment.

Management

Stone dissolution is unlikely to be successful so conservative management is not indicated. Cystoscopic crushing of the calculus (*litholapaxy*), using an *optical lithotrite*, can be combined with resection of the prostate or bladder neck, but has a complication rate of up to 25%; complications are usually related to bladder perforation. Litholapaxy may be impossible if the stone is very large and cannot be grasped in the jaws of the optical lithotrite. Cystoscopic lithotripsy using electrohydraulic, ultrasonic, ballistic or laser fragmentation is safer but may be ineffective if the calculus is very hard. For very large or very hard calculi, open surgical removal by *cystolithotomy* or by percutaneous extraction may be necessary. Extracorporeal shock wave lithotripsy (ESWL) is ineffective, often leaves fragments within the bladder and usually requires multiple treatments.

Prevention of recurrent bladder calculi requires elimination of infection and treatment of the underlying cause, usually bladder outflow obstruction due to prostatic enlargement.

Calculi in bladders augmented with bowel segments

Up to 20% of patients who have undergone augmentation cystoplasty using an isolated segment of bowel develop bladder calculi. The commonest causes are urinary infection, excess mucus production, hypocitraturia and foreign bodies or sutures within the bladder. They may be managed cystoscopically but occasionally require open surgical removal.

Urethral calculi in men

Calculi rarely form de novo in the urethra, except proximal to a urethral stricture or within a urethral diverticulum; the

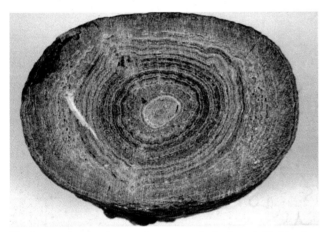

Fig. 1 Large, laminated, **ammonium urate calculus** from the bladder of a child.

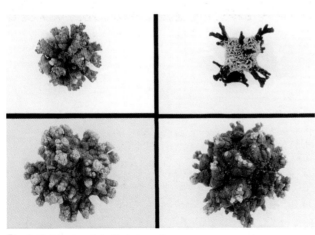

Fig. 2 **Calcium oxalate 'jackstones'.**

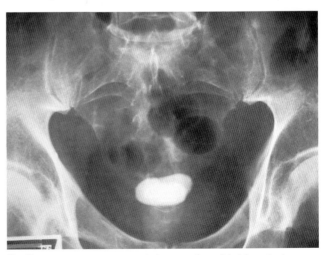

Fig. 3 Plain abdominal radiograph showing a **large bladder calculus.**

majority arise from the upper tracts or the bladder and are voided into the urethra.

Clinical features

There is usually pain in the urethra on voiding with sudden stoppage and dribbling of urine. The calculus may be palpable in the penile or bulbar urethra and may be visible if it lies close to the urethral meatus. The diagnosis can be confirmed by plain abdominal radiograph, urethral ultrasound or cystourethroscopy.

Management

Anterior calculi can be removed under direct vision with forceps or with stone baskets. Direct incision into the urethra may be necessary for calculi in the penile urethra. Calculi in the more proximal urethra can often be dislodged into the bladder and managed as bladder calculi.

Prostatic calculi

Prostatic calculi are common in men over 50 years. They are usually asymptomatic and occur in clusters, associated with benign prostatic hyperplasia or carcinoma of the prostate. They form as a result of duct obstruction and stasis of prostatic fluid, and represent calcified corpora amylacea trapped between the central adenoma of the prostate and the prostatic capsule. Prostatic calculi are commonly seen incidentally on abdominal radiograph (Fig. 4), abdominal ultrasound, CT or during transrectal prostatic ultrasound.

Management

No specific treatment is needed, but prostatic calculi are usually released during transurethral resection of the prostate once the prostatic capsule is reached.

Urethral calculi in women

Calculi in the normal female urethra are very rare. Occasionally, they may occur in a urethral diverticulum (Fig. 5) as a result of urinary stasis and infection.

Clinical features

Symptoms are usually due to urinary tract infection, but pain during coitus with leakage of urine and a purulent introital discharge are diagnostic. There is usually a palpable mass in the anterior vaginal wall, and pus or urine can be expressed from the urethra by pressure on the mass. Diagnosis is by cystourethrography or transvaginal urethral ultrasound.

Management

Definitive treatment involves local excision of the diverticulum via an incision in the anterior vaginal wall with direct removal of the intact calculus.

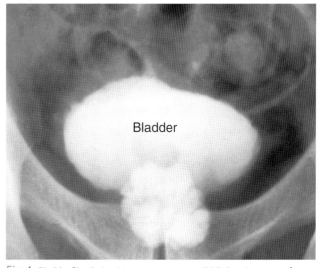

Fig. 4 Bladder film during intravenous urogram (IVU) showing **extensive prostatic calcification.**

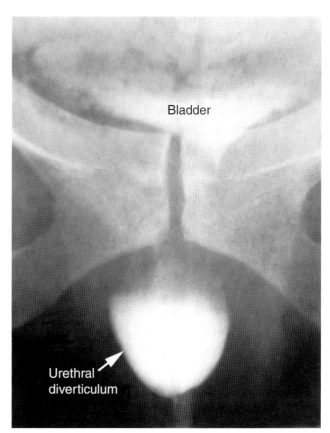

Fig. 5 Cystogram showing a **large urethral diverticulum** in a female.

> ### Key points
>
> ■ Bladder calculi usually form de novo within the bladder as a result of prostatic enlargement.
>
> ■ Surgical treatment by litholapaxy or cystolithotripsy is the most effective treatment but usually needs to be combined with treatment for the underlying bladder outflow obstruction.
>
> ■ Urethral calculi are rare and normally form in the bladder or upper tracts, except in women where they form in a urethral diverticulum.

Upper Tract Obstruction

Nephrological Disorders

Renal failure

Acute renal failure

Acute renal failure (ARF) is a sudden drop in renal function characterised by failure to maintain electrolyte and fluid homeostasis; it implies a rise in serum creatinine of $>50\%$ over baseline levels or a decrease in creatinine clearance by $>50\%$ associated with oliguria ($<400\,mL/24\,h$) or anuria. It is caused by prerenal, renal or post-renal factors (Fig. 1).

Clinical features

The diagnosis is usually made from the history, the presence of oliguria or anuria and the plasma biochemical findings (uraemia, acidosis, hyperkalaemia and raised serum creatinine); urine biochemistry may help to determine the type of ARF (Table 1). A plain abdominal radiograph excludes calculi, and an ultrasound will detect the presence of obstructive uropathy or hereditary renal cystic disease. Computerised tomography (CT), retrograde pyelography or antegrade pyelography may be necessary to assess the site of any obstruction. Radionuclide renography helps to assess arterial flow to the kidneys.

Prerenal ARF

This is due to hypoperfusion of the kidneys, which causes release of noradrenaline and angiotensin, renal vasoconstriction and decreased glomerular filtration rate (GFR). The main differential diagnosis is retention of urine (excluded by ultrasound or urethral catheterisation) and hypovolaemia (which responds to an intravenous fluid load).

Renal ARF

This is usually caused by glomerulonephritis, interstitial nephritis or acute tubular necrosis (ATN). Glomerulonephritis results in proteinuria, haematuria and red cell casts in the urine; interstitial nephritis causes sterile pyuria, white cell casts and eosinophiluria, and may be caused by nephrotoxic drugs. ATN is a severe form of renal ARF that has a high mortality (30–80%) and is caused by adenosine triphosphate (ATP) depletion in the kidney with a profound fall in renal blood flow, especially in the outer medulla. The oliguric phase of ATN begins within 24 h of the hypoperfusion insult and lasts up to 4 days. As renal function recovers, a diuretic phase ensues when large losses of electrolytes and fluid can occur, resulting in 25% of the deaths due to ATN. Finally, there is a recovery phase, which may take 3–12 months for renal function to stabilise.

Post-renal ARF

This is due to bilateral obstruction, but can occur in unilateral obstruction if there is pre-existing dysfunction in the contralateral kidney. There is often a history of pain with haematuria and

Table 1 Urinary findings in acute renal failure			
Type	Urinary sodium (mmol/L)	Urinary osmolarity (mOsm)	Urine/plasma creatinine ratio
Prerenal	< 20	> 500	> 20
Renal	> 40	< 300	< 20
Post-renal			
Acute	< 20	> 500	> 20
Chronic	< 40	> 350	< 20

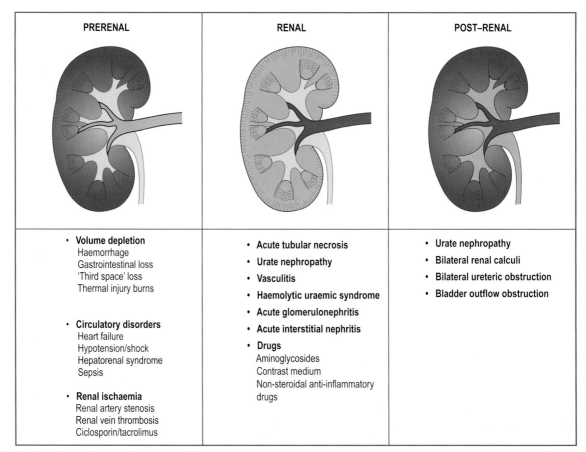

PRERENAL	RENAL	POST–RENAL
• **Volume depletion** Haemorrhage Gastrointestinal loss 'Third space' loss Thermal injury burns • **Circulatory disorders** Heart failure Hypotension/shock Hepatorenal syndrome Sepsis • **Renal ischaemia** Renal artery stenosis Renal vein thrombosis Ciclosporin/tacrolimus	• **Acute tubular necrosis** • **Urate nephropathy** • **Vasculitis** • **Haemolytic uraemic syndrome** • **Acute glomerulonephritis** • **Acute interstitial nephritis** • **Drugs** Aminoglycosides Contrast medium Non-steroidal anti-inflammatory drugs	• **Urate nephropathy** • **Bilateral renal calculi** • **Bilateral ureteric obstruction** • **Bladder outflow obstruction**

Fig. 1 **Classification and causes of acute renal failure.**

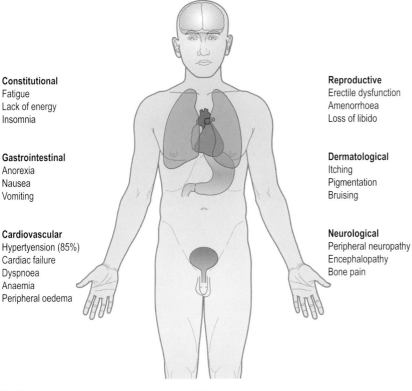

Constitutional
Fatigue
Lack of energy
Insomnia

Gastrointestinal
Anorexia
Nausea
Vomiting

Cardiovascular
Hypertyension (85%)
Cardiac failure
Dyspnoea
Anaemia
Peripheral oedema

Reproductive
Erectile dysfunction
Amenorrhoea
Loss of libido

Dermatological
Itching
Pigmentation
Bruising

Neurological
Peripheral neuropathy
Encephalopathy
Bone pain

Fig. 2 **Signs and symptoms of chronic renal failure.**

Table 2 **Indications for dialysis in acute renal failure**	
Indication	**Signs**
Intractable volume overload	Pulmonary oedema
Acidosis	Serum bicarbonate < 12 mmol/L or arterial pH < 7.15
Hyperkalaemia	Serum potassium > 7 mmol/L
Uraemic pericarditis	Cardiac failure with pericardial friction rub
Uraemic symptoms	Urea rising by > 16 mmol/day or by > 35 mmol/L

Table 3 **Causes (%) of chronic renal failure (CRF) and endstage renal disease (ESRD)**	
Diabetes mellitus	34
Hypertensive nephrosclerosis	29
Chronic glomerulonephritis	13
Unclear	10
Others	6
Interstitial glomerulonephritis	
Chronic pyelonephritis	
Obstructive nephropathy	5
Hereditary cystic disease	3

evidence of previous abdominal surgery, stones, malignancy or radiotherapy.

Management of ARF

Treatment depends on the cause. In ATN, loop diuretics, mannitol and dopamine infusions may reduce renal damage by speeding transfer from the oliguric to the diuretic phase. The aim is to optimise volume status by balancing fluid input against total output plus an allowance for insensible loss. Calorific support is needed with adequate carbohydrates, and protein intake should be reduced. Secondary infection contributes significantly to mortality, and erosive gastritis needs to be prevented using H2-receptor anatagonists (cimetidine, ranitidine). The main clinical concern is hyperkalaemia (>7 mmol/L); this can be managed by glucose–insulin infusions or by ion-exchange resins, but haemodialysis, haemofiltration or peritoneal dialysis may be needed for this and other specific situations (Table 2).

Chronic renal failure

This is defined as kidney damage or a reduction in GFR to <60 mL/min for more than 3 months. Diabetes mellitus is the commonest cause (Table 3). Clinical features are varied and affect many body systems (Fig. 2).

Management

Medical management is aimed at preventing or delaying progression to endstage renal disease (ESRD) and should be under the supervision of a nephrologist. Control of diabetes mellitus must be optimised. Anaemia (normochromic normocytic) is best treated with recombinant human erythropoietin; blood transfusions carry the risk of sensitisation to antigens, which jeopardises the survival of a future renal transplant. Hypertension accelerates the loss of renal function and should be treated appropriately with angiotensin-converting enzyme (ACE) inhibitors (ramipril). Restriction of protein (to 0.6 g/kg day), potassium (to 40 mmol/day), sodium and fluid intake is beneficial. Acidosis may require treatment with oral bicarbonate, and renal osteodystrophy is treated by correcting hyperphosphataemia and hypocalcaemia. Coagulopathy with poor platelet function may respond to treatment with fresh frozen plasma and desmopressin (DDAVP).

Progression to ESRD is most likely in older patients and those with cardiovascular disease, diabetes mellitus and poor nutritional status.

Endstage renal disease

The onset of endstage renal disease is difficult to define, but most nephrologists accept a GFR of <15 mL/min as the cut-off point at which simple conservative management is no longer effective. Once this stage is reached, renal replacement therapy is required by haemodialysis, peritoneal dialysis or renal transplantation. Dialysis may be required at an earlier stage in patients with uncontrolled hypertension, symptomatic uraemia (especially when associated with pericarditis, mental changes, nausea and vomiting), severe hyperkalaemia, volume overload, severe coagulopathy, severe acidosis and neuropathy. The ultimate aim is a renal transplant, which provides the best quality of life, but the limited availability of kidneys for transplantation means that some patients will remain on dialysis for their entire lives.

> ### Key points
>
> ■ Acute renal failure may be due to prerenal, renal or post-renal causes.
>
> ■ Management is usually conservative with dialysis reserved for specific situations in which medical measures fail to control electrolyte and fluid homeostasis.
>
> ■ Acute tubular necrosis has a particularly poor prognosis and a high mortality.
>
> ■ Chronic renal failure is most commonly due to diabetes mellitus and is managed by medical means to slow the progression to endstage renal disease.
>
> ■ Dialysis is necessary once endstage renal disease has occurred, but the ultimate aim is renal transplantation.

Dialysis and transplantation

Haemodialysis

Haemodialysis requires access to the circulation using a tunnelled double-lumen venous cannula, a peripheral vascular graft between the arterial and venous system or an arteriovenous fistula in the non-dominant arm (*Cimino fistula*). Venous cannulae allow immediate haemodialysis, but a peripheral fistula requires 4–6 weeks to mature before it can be used for vascular access. The process requires the use of a dialysis machine (Fig. 1), which filters arterial blood from the circulation across a semipermeable membrane and returns the blood to the venous system. Haemodialysis is usually performed three times per week with each session taking 4 h to complete.

No equipment is required at home, and it provides good support for the patient but does require regular hospital visits, permanent vascular access and needle puncture for each treatment. Problems with vascular access may occur together with disequilibrium (due to the dehydrating effect of removing urea), hypotension (in up to 50% of treatments), muscle cramps and arrhythmias. Acquired renal cystic disease develops in 60–80% of patients undergoing haemodialysis for more than 3 years.

Haemofiltration provides a more rapid means of improving fluid and electrolyte balance with the ability to filter large volumes over a short period of time. It is often used in emergency situations for acute renal failure but is rarely employed routinely in endstage renal disease.

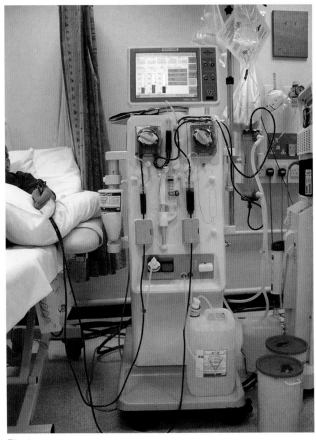

Fig. 1 **Dialysis machine.**

Peritoneal dialysis

Peritoneal dialysis is safer than haemodialysis and has fewer complications, but is contraindicated in patients with peritoneal fibrosis, intestinal stomas, abdominal hernias, obesity, prosthetic heart valves and hereditary cystic disease. A long-term catheter (*Tenckhoff catheter*) is inserted through the abdominal wall by laparoscopy or open surgery and provides access to the peritoneal cavity. The large surface area of the peritoneal cavity is utilised to filter waste products by running dialysis fluid into the abdomen and allowing it to drain (Fig. 2).

Continuous ambulatory peritoneal dialysis (CAPD) is performed throughout the day with 1.5–3 L being used for each exchange; the dialysate is emptied four times a day and replaced manually with new fluid. *Automated peritoneal dialysis* (APD) is performed at night by a machine which exchanges 8–12 L over 10 h, leaving 1–2 L in the peritoneal cavity during the day

CAPD and APD mean fewer hospital visits, less need for venepuncture and few dietary restrictions. Mechanical problems (pain, leakage, poor flow and scrotal oedema) are rare. The main hazard of peritoneal dialysis is the risk of *peritonitis*. Most infections are caused by staphylococci, but fungal and mycobacterial infections are also seen. Treatment is by rapid flushes of dialysate, intraperitoneal antibiotics and broad-spectrum oral antibiotics. Infection with *Pseudomonas* or fungi are indications for removal of the dialysis catheter.

Renal transplantation

All patients should undergo a full physical and psychological assessment before transplantation. Full biochemical screening is important together with ABO blood grouping and tissue typing. Urological assessment (cystography, cystoscopy and urodynamic studies) is necessary in patients with lower urinary tract symptoms. Sepsis, acquired immunodeficiency syndrome (AIDS), active hepatitis, impaired mental function, tuberculosis and active malignancy are contraindications to renal transplantation; patients with a past history of malignancy can receive a transplant after a 3- to 5-year recurrence-free period. Preliminary removal of the native kidneys may be required in polycystic kidney disease, uncontrolled hypertension and in patients with obstructive nephropathy or renal calculi.

Cadaveric donation is the main source of kidneys for transplantation. The donor must also undergo detailed tests of serology, blood grouping and histocompatibility; donor kidneys are usually removed en bloc (with arteries, veins and ureter carefully preserved) and are treated with cold perfusion before being packed in ice for transportation. Living related donors require detailed assessment of the renal vasculature before nephrectomy, and donor operations are now frequently performed laparoscopically to minimise morbidity.

Histocompatibility is determined by ABO blood grouping and by assessing human leucocyte antigens (HLAs). The major histocompatibility complex (MHC) is a cluster of genes on the short arm of chromosome 6. The cell surface

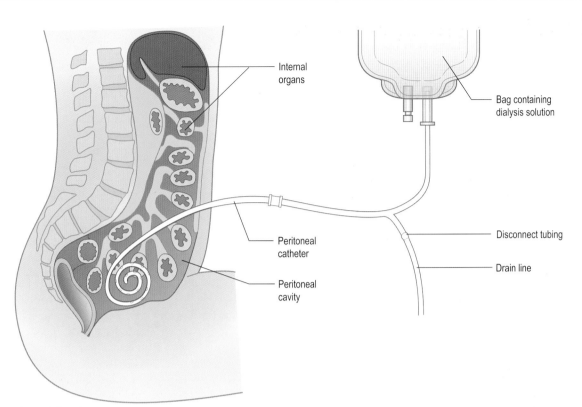

Internal organs

Bag containing dialysis solution

Peritoneal catheter

Disconnect tubing

Drain line

Peritoneal cavity

Fig. 2 **Peritoneal dialysis.**

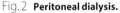

Table 1	**Immunosuppression following renal transplantation**
Polyclonal/monoclonal antibodies	
Muromanab-CD3 (OKT3)	
Calcineurin inhibitors	
Ciclosporin A	
Tacrolimus	
Purine synthesis inhibitors	
Azathioprine, cyclophosphamide	
Methotrexate, mycophenolate	
Steroids	

Table 2	**Complications of renal transplantation**
Vascular	Seen in 6–30% of patients
	Renal artery stenosis may be iatrogenic or due to atherosclerosis (requiring exploration or balloon angioplasty)
	Renal vein thrombosis (in less than 1%) results in graft loss
Urological	Anastomotic leakage (3–10%) or obstruction may respond to drainage and stenting
	Lymphocele may cause late obstruction (1–18%)
	Bladder leakage usually responds to prolonged catheterisation
Infection	Opportunistic infections arise 1–6 months after surgery
	Viral warts occur in 50% of patients
	Fungal infections
Rejection	Hyperacute (accelerated)
	Acute
	Chronic
Hypertension	Seen in up to 80%
	12% develop renal artery stenosis
Malignancy	Lymphoma (1–2%), usually non-Hodgkin's B-cell lymphoma
	Skin cancers are 20 times more common than normal

markers are HLAs, with antigens in the A, B and DR locus being most important in histocompatibility; the greater the antigenic match, the greater the likelihood of graft survival.

Renal transplantation is normally performed into an extraperitoneal site with anastomosis of the renal vessels to the patient's internal iliac artery and external iliac vein; the ureter is anastomosed directly to the bladder over a ureteric stent. Post-operative fluid management is critical, and patients should receive low-dose anticoagulation to prevent venous thrombosis. Immunosuppression should be commenced immediately (Table 1); most patients require a combination of a calcineurin inhibitor (*tacrolimus* or *ciclosporin*), azathioprine and steroids initially. Doppler ultrasound or ^{99m}Tc-mercaptoacetyltriglycine (MAG3) scintigraphy is performed in the early postoperative period to assess transplant perfusion.

The major complications of renal transplantation are shown in Table 2. Successful renal transplantation offers good quality of life without the need for dialysis. Men may regain reproductive function, and women often restart menstruation and are able to conceive.

Key points

■ Haemodialysis provides good renal replacement therapy but ties patients to hospital visits and fixed schedules.

■ Peritoneal dialysis offers patients more freedom from hospital visits and is generally well tolerated.

■ Renal transplantation provides good quality of life, and research into new immunosuppressive regimes offers further improvement in the outlook for these patients.

Renal and adrenal hypertension

Hypertension is defined as a systolic blood pressure >160 mmHg, a diastolic blood pressure >95 mmHg or a combination of both. In most hypertensive patients, there is no specific underlying cause (*essential hypertension*), but a small proportion of patients have *secondary hypertension* with a recognisable renal or endocrine cause.

Certain features of hypertension should raise the suspicion of a secondary cause (Table 1). Urologists contribute to the management of renal parenchymal hypertension, Cushing syndrome, Conn syndrome, phaeochromocytoma and renovascular hypertension.

Renal parenchymal hypertension

This is seen in chronic pyelonephritis, hydronephrosis, segmental renal hypoplasia (Ask-Upmark kidney) and vesicoureteric reflux, usually in unilateral cases. Control of the hypertension by nephrectomy may be effective but only if the contralateral kidney has not already suffered irreversible hypertensive changes. Some renal tumours (e.g. adenocarcinoma, nephroblastoma and juxtaglomerular tumours) may cause secondary hypertension, which can be resolved by nephrectomy.

Cushing syndrome

Cushing syndrome is usually steroid induced. In patients not receiving steroids, 80% have Cushing's disease (due to a pituitary adenoma) and 20% have inappropriate adrenocorticotrophic hormone (ACTH) secretion (due to an adrenal adenoma or ectopic ACTH production).

Clinical diagnosis (Fig. 1)
Plasma cortisol levels are raised with loss of normal circadian rhythm, and urinary excretion of free cortisol, 17-oxogenic steroids and 17-oxosteroids is raised. Plasma ACTH levels may be raised, and the normal plasma cortisol rise in response to insulin-induced hypoglycaemia is absent. Skull radiograph may show expansion of the pituitary fossa, and localisation of an adrenal tumour can be accomplished using ^{131}I-iodocholesterol scintigraphy, computerised tomography (CT) or magnetic resonance imaging (MRI).

Treatment
Bilateral adrenalectomy is indicated only if a pituitary tumour cannot be identified; it is normally performed laparoscopically. Steroid replacement is necessary after surgery, and 10–20% of patients subsequently develop a pituitary tumour (*Nelson*

syndrome). Functioning adrenal adenomas should also be excised laparoscopically, but incidental, non-functioning adrenal adenomas, seen in 10–15% of the population, do not cause Cushing's disease. The prognosis of malignant adrenal tumours is poor.

Conn syndrome and primary hyperaldosteronism

Seventy per cent of patients with primary hyperaldosteronism have an aldosterone-producing tumour arising from the zona glomerulosa of the adrenal gland (*Conn syndrome*); the remainder have idiopathic, bilateral adrenal hyperplasia.

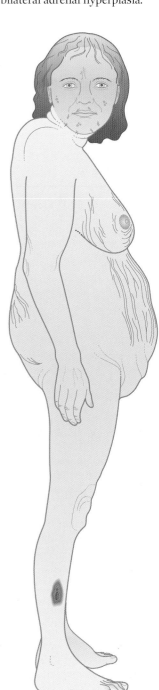

- Upper body obesity with thin arms and legs
- Buffalo hump
- Red, round face
- High blood sugar
- High blood pressure
- Vertigo
- Blurry vision
- Acne
- Female balding
- Water retention
- Menstrual irregularities
- Thin skin and bruising
- Purple striae
- Poor wound healing
- Hirsutism
- Severe depression
- Congnitive difficulties
- Emotional instability
- Sleep disorders
- Fatigue

Table 1 **Factors suggesting a diagnosis of secondary hypertension**
Age of onset < 30 years or > 55 years
Strong family history of hypertension
Sudden onset and short duration
Accelerated hypertension
Hypertension difficult to control with drugs
Epigastric bruit (systolic and diastolic)
Hypertensive retinopathy (grade II or more)

Fig. 1 **Clinical features of Cushing syndrome.**

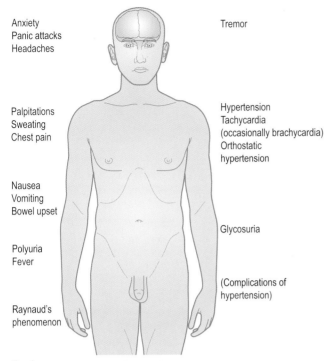

Anxiety
Panic attacks
Headaches

Tremor

Palpitations
Sweating
Chest pain

Hypertension
Tachycardia
(occasionally brachycardia)
Orthostatic
hypertension

Nausea
Vomiting
Bowel upset

Glycosuria

Polyuria
Fever

(Complications of
hypertension)

Raynaud's
phenomenon

Fig. 2 **Clinical features of phaeochromocytoma.**

Table 2 **The causes of renovascular hypertension**	
Atherosclerosis	70%
Idiopathic	>25%
Intimal fibroplasia (10%)	
Fibromuscular hyperplasia (2–3%)	
Medial fibroplasia (75–80%)	
Subadventitial fibroplasia (10–15%)	
Other abnormalities	<5%
Renal artery aneurysm	
Arteriovenous fistula	

Clinical diagnosis

Conn syndrome usually presents in young women as severe hypertension associated with muscle weakness, tetany, nocturia and constipation. Adrenal venography with measurement of venous aldosterone levels is diagnostic, and radionuclide scintigraphy with ^{131}I-iodocholesterol may help in locating small tumours. Adrenal adenoma and hyperplasia can be distinguished by the plasma aldosterone response to postural change; levels fall in the erect position with adenomas but rise with hyperplasia.

Treatment

Treatment for Conn syndrome is surgical removal of the adrenal adenoma or hyperplastic glands. Laparoscopic excision is preferred to open surgery because of its lower morbidity and mortality. Surgery cures the hypertension is 60% of patients with an adrenal adenoma. In bilateral adrenal hyperplasia, surgery cures only 30%. Long-term treatment with spironolactone (100–400 mg/day) or amiloride (10–40 mg/day) is used to control hypertension if surgical treatment fails.

Phaeochromocytoma

This is usually a tumour of the renal medulla that secretes catecholamines (adrenaline and noradrenaline). Hypertension is episodic in 33% of patients with intermittent periods of normotension. Ten per cent of tumours are malignant, 10% multiple, 10% bilateral and 10% extra-adrenal, while some cases are associated with multiple endocrine adenomatosis.

Clinical diagnosis (Fig. 2)

Diagnosis is confirmed by finding raised plasma levels of catecholamines and raised metabolite levels (vanillylmandelic acid, VMA) in the urine. ^{131}I-meta-iodobenzylguanidine scintigraphy may help to localise extra-adrenal tumours, but CT and MRI are more reliable.

Treatment

Surgical excision (open or laparoscopic) is invariably curative, but operative handling of the tumour can precipitate acute hypertension due to massive catecholamine release; this can be prevented by intraoperative administration of α-blockers, β-blockers and vasodilators.

Renovascular hypertension

Renovascular hypertension is most commonly due to atherosclerotic obstruction of the renal artery (Table 2) and should be suspected if there is an audible epigastric bruit.

Clinical diagnosis

Intravenous urogram (IVU) shows an indistinct nephrogram in the affected kidney with a delayed pyelogram, notching of the collecting system by collateral vessels and a size disparity of >1.5 cm between the kidneys. Selective renal vein renin sampling is relatively unreliable. Renal scintigraphy (with ^{99m}Tc-mercaptoacetyltriglycine, MAG3) following the administration of captopril shows delayed isotope uptake, asymmetrical peaking, cortical retention and a reduction in glomerular filtration rate with a 90% sensitivity for renal artery stenosis. Angiography using contrast medium, CT or MRI is the definitive investigation.

Treatment

Surgical reconstruction, angioplasty or autotransplantation of the kidney have a 50–60% cure rate for atherosclerotic renovascular hypertension; angioplasty in atherosclerotic obstruction has a restenosis rate of 10–35%. For idiopathic renal artery stenosis, angioplasty or endovascular stenting produces the best results with cure rates of over 90%. Renal artery aneurysms or arteriovenous fistulae may require surgical repair or embolisation.

Key points

- Secondary hypertension is rare but should be suspected in young patients, when hypertension is severe or difficult to control, when there is a strong family history and when there is an epigastric bruit.

- Renal parenchymal hypertension responds to surgery only if the contralateral kidney is unaffected by hypertensive changes.

- Endocrine hypertension is usually caused by oral contraceptive agents, but adrenal or pituitary tumours may be implicated and respond well to surgical treatment.

- Renovascular hypertension is usually due to atherosclerosis, which has a tendency to recur or progress after surgical reconstruction.

- Percutaneous transluminal angioplasty produces the best results for non-atherosclerotic renal artery stenosis.

Lower Urinary Tract Obstruction

Pathophysiology and assessment

Bladder outlet obstruction (BOO) may be produced by any infravesical abnormality such as urethral stricture or stenosis of the external meatus but, in the ageing male, it is usually due to prostatic enlargement; whatever the cause, the symptoms are usually similar.

Clinical features

The symptoms associated with BOO are shown in Table 1 and are collectively known by the descriptive term lower urinary tract symptoms (LUTS).

Benign prostatic hyperplasia (BPH) is ubiquitous in the ageing male, becoming evident from the age of 50 years. BPH occurs primarily in the transition zone of the prostate, through which the urethra passes, resulting in enlargement of the glandular tissue of the prostate. Increased tone within the smooth muscle of the prostatic stroma and bladder neck also occurs, resulting in increased resistance and consequent BOO. The three entities of LUTS, BPH and BOO are independent variables, but may coexist and determine the clinical situation (Fig. 1).

BOO has dynamic and static components. The dynamic component is due to increased tone within the smooth muscle of prostatic stroma, periurethral and bladder neck regions (under alpha-adrenergic neuronal control). The static component comprises enlargement of the glandular component of the prostate, which causes a physical narrowing of the urethra. The relative influence of these varies between patients and in individual patients at different times.

BOO is a physiological abnormality, which can be confirmed by pressure flow (urodynamic) studies demonstrating that the pressure in the bladder is >60 cm of water and that the urinary flow rate is reduced (Fig. 2). The use of computer-generated nomograms allows categorisation of patients into obstructed, equivocal or non-obstructed (Fig. 3).

In response to the obstructive process, the detrusor muscle within the bladder undergoes a change in its physical characteristics (detrusor hypertrophy) and in its function; alterations in the nerve supply result in *denervation supersensitivity*. This causes secondary detrusor instability (DI) and is responsible for the storage symptoms shown in Table 1. Primary DI, without obstruction, may also cause LUTS, but must be differentiated from secondary DI because treatment is different. Age-related changes within the bladder wall may compound and distort the effects of BOO; the detrusor muscle acquires increased amounts of fibrous tissue, resulting in reduced compliance and impaired contractility.

Assessment

Before treatment can be instituted, patients with LUTS suggestive of BOO need assessment to determine whether obstruction is actually present. The underlying cause, whether benign prostatic hypertrophy, carcinoma of the prostate or a urethral stricture, also needs to be determined. Assessment involves taking a careful history and using the International Prostate Symptom Score (I-PSS; see Appendix, p. 151), in which the LUTS are scored together with a quality of life (or bother) score. Incontinence, retention of urine, urinary

Table 1 **Lower urinary tract symptoms (LUTS)**	
Voiding (obstructive) symptoms	**Storage (irritative) symptoms**
Hesitancy	Frequency
Poor flow	Nocturia
Terminal dribbling	Urgency
Incomplete bladder emptying	Urge incontinence
Straining to void	

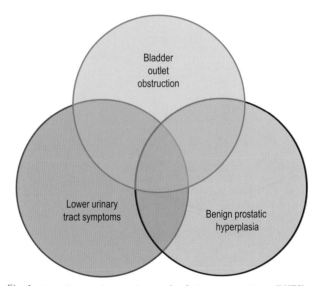

Fig. 1 Venn diagram showing the **overlap between symptoms (LUTS), histopathology (BPH) and pathophysiology (BOO).**

infection, chronic renal failure and haematuria should also be addressed individually and, if found to be secondary to BOO, may influence treatment decisions.

Examination should include the abdomen (for an enlarged bladder), the genitalia and digital rectal examination (DRE) to determine the shape, size and consistency of the prostate. At the same time, an assessment of perianal sensation and tone can be made. Urinalysis should be performed for signs of infection or haematuria. A frequency–volume chart (see Appendix, p. 149) should be completed by the patient to assess functional bladder capacity and to seek evidence of nocturnal polyuria, which is usually due to poor water handling at night in association with ageing kidneys and will not respond to the standard treatment for BOO.

Biochemical investigations include serum electrolytes, creatinine and prostate-specific antigen (PSA) once the patient has been counselled about the limitations of PSA testing and the consequences of identifying an abnormal result. PSA is also useful as a surrogate marker of prostatic size and, if >1.4 ng/mL, there is a greater risk of progressive symptoms.

Patients should perform a simple urinary flow rate and, after completion of voiding, the post-micturition residual volume of urine within the bladder should be measured using ultrasound. From these preliminary studies, it is possible to identify the majority of patients with BOO without resort to further investigation. The likelihood of BOO with a peak urinary flow <10 mL/s is 90%, with 10–15 mL/s is 50% and with >15 mL/s is 30%, provided at least 150 mL of urine have been passed during the study. When the diagnosis of BOO is unclear or storage symptoms predominate, formal urodynamic studies may be indicated.

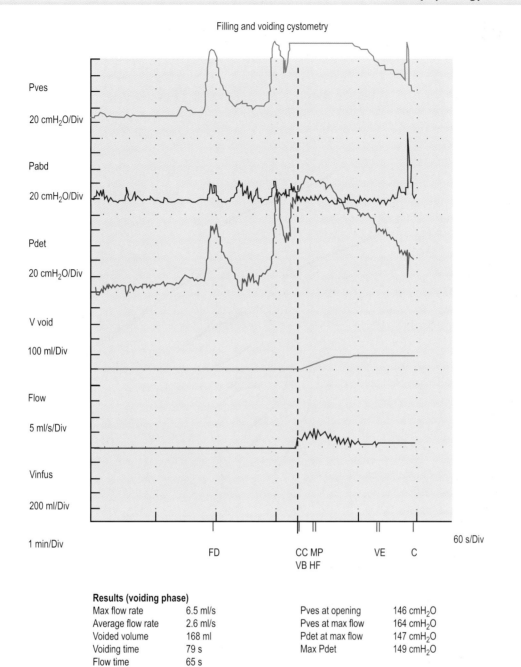

Filling and voiding cystometry

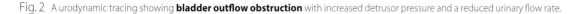

Results (voiding phase)

Max flow rate	6.5 ml/s	Pves at opening	146 cmH$_2$O
Average flow rate	2.6 ml/s	Pves at max flow	164 cmH$_2$O
Voided volume	168 ml	Pdet at max flow	147 cmH$_2$O
Voiding time	79 s	Max Pdet	149 cmH$_2$O
Flow time	65 s		
Time to max flow	8 s		

Fig. 2 A urodynamic tracing showing **bladder outflow obstruction** with increased detrusor pressure and a reduced urinary flow rate.

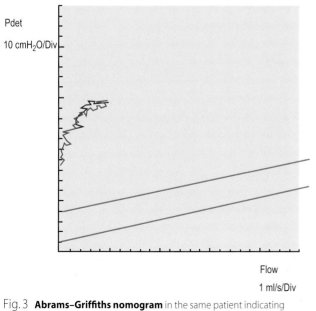

Fig. 3 **Abrams–Griffiths nomogram** in the same patient indicating bladder outlet obstruction.

> ## Key points
>
> ■ Bladder outlet obstruction (BOO) is a urodynamic definition of raised detrusor pressure (60 cm of water) in response to increased bladder outlet resistance.
>
> ■ The commonest cause in the ageing male is benign prostatic hyperplasia (BPH), but any condition that reduces the calibre of the urinary tract at or below the bladder neck may contribute.
>
> ■ The term lower urinary tract symptoms (LUTS) is a descriptive one, and LUTS are not synonymous with BOO.
>
> ■ LUTS, BPH and BOO may exist in isolation or in combination.
>
> ■ Clinical assessment involves the quantification of symptoms and determination of the urinary flow together with the efficiency of bladder emptying.

Benign prostatic hyperplasia

The term benign prostatic hyperplasia (BPH) refers to a specific histopathological abnormality of stromal and epithelial hyperplasia, which, according to autopsy studies, becomes increasingly common with advancing age. BPH is usually identified clinically by digital rectal examination (DRE). However, a pathological diagnosis of BPH can be confirmed only after histological analysis (Fig. 1). BPH is not present in men under the age of 30 years, but prostatic growth due to BPH starts to become evident in the fourth decade. This process begins as diffuse hyperplasia, later progressing to nodule development (Fig. 2), which becomes apparent by the fifth decade. By the age of 85 years, 90% of men will have evidence of microscopic BPH. The rate of prostatic growth is approximately 2% by volume per year in men between the age of 55 and 75 years; racial and environmental issues have a significant influence on growth rate.

Zonal anatomy of the prostate

The zonal anatomy of the prostate was described on pp. 8 and 9. The transition zone surrounds the urethra and is itself surrounded by the central zone; this is perforated by the ejaculatory ducts, emerging from the conjoined seminal vesicles and vas deferens to open into the floor of the urethra at the level of the verumontanum. Surrounding both the transition and the central zones is the peripheral zone, which is the part of the prostate palpable on DRE.

In young men, the peripheral zone is the largest but, as BPH develops almost exclusively in the transition zone, this becomes the zone of largest volume in the ageing prostate.

Aetiology of benign prostatic hyperplasia

The established factors necessary for the development of BPH are advancing age and the presence of functioning testes. Testosterone produced in the testes is activated within the prostate by an enzyme (5α-reductase) on the nuclear membrane. This results in the production of dihydrotestosterone (DHT); DHT binds to androgen receptors to form complexes, which then associate with the genome. This pathological process is influenced by both androgens and estrogens as well as by the action of growth factors, which either stimulate or inhibit growth. Delicate changes within this hormonal milieu can have a significant impact on prostate growth.

Intrinsic regulation of prostatic growth

The prostate can be regarded as having both epithelial and stromal components. These are separated by a basement membrane in which the basal cells abut the luminal cell population. Scattered between these cellular components are neuroendocrine cells. The prostatic stroma comprises a complex of different cell types surrounded by extracellular matrix. The stroma plays a major part in the induction and control of prostatic growth. Prostatic growth is dependent on the balance between many factors (Table 1).

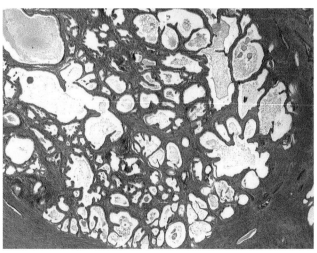

Fig. 1 **Microscopic appearances of BPH.**

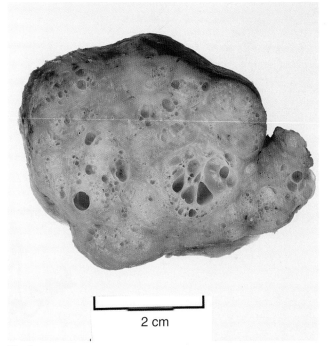

2 cm

Fig. 2 Gross pathology showing **nodule development in BPH.**

Table 1 **Factors regulating prostatic growth**	
Extrinsic	**Intrinsic**
Testis	Epithelium
Androgens	Luminal cells
Estrogens	Basal cells
Non-androgenic factors	Neuroendocrine cells
Environmental	Stroma
Diet	Fibroblasts
Micro-organisms	Smooth muscle cells
	Extracellular matrix
Urethra	Genetic
Urine	Hereditary conditions
Seminal fluid	Homeobox genes
	Other
	Endocrine organs
	Neurotransmitters
	Immunological factors

The growth factors produced within the prostate are proteins that can exert an effect on cells via an autocrine, paracrine or intracrine effect. There are a large number of growth factors, but epidermal growth factor (EGF), fibroblast growth factor (FGF2) and insulin-like growth factor (IGF-1) are responsible for 80% of the positive modulating growth effects. In conjunction with androgens, these growth factors work together to maintain normal prostatic growth. The major inhibitory growth factor is transforming growth factor (TGF-β). This exerts a different action on epithelial and stromal cells, but its main role is to regulate smooth muscle differentiation rather than balancing proliferation and apoptosis (programmed cell death).

Extrinsic factors

The most influential extrinsic factor is the testis itself, which produces androgens, estrogens and non-androgenic testicular factors. The most important androgen, testosterone, is converted to the highly potent dihydrotestosterone (DHT) by 5α-reductase, and DHT results in nuclear signalling with the production of intrinsic growth factors that ultimately mediate androgen action. Estrogens cause proliferation of the stromal cells and the inhibition of prostatic epithelium. With increasing age, the ratio of estrogens to DHT within the prostate increases to a greater extent than that seen in the circulation. A number of extratesticular hormones, especially prolactin, have the capacity to modify the signalling process between epithelial and stromal cells within the prostate; neurotransmitters and neurotrophins also influence this stromal–epithelial interaction.

A number of environmental factors, including prostatic inflammation and diet, exert an inhibitory effect on prostatic growth. Dietary influences such as the ingestion of plant estrogens (*phytoestrogens*) play a major role in Asian and Oriental men who tend to have smaller prostates and a lower incidence of BPH.

The genetic elements of BPH are unclear, but the development of large prostates at a young age in some families suggests a possible genetic influence, although the exact causative mechanisms are unclear.

Key points

- Benign prostatic hyperplasia becomes evident in the fourth decade and is present in 90% of men aged 85 years.
- Benign prostatic hyperplasia arises in the transition zone, and this develops into the largest zone with increasing age.
- Advancing age and functioning testes are prerequisites for BPH.
- Prostatic growth is a balance between intrinsic and extrinsic factors.
- Intrinsic factors govern the interactions between stromal and epithelial compartments within the prostate.

Acute urinary retention

Acute retention of urine (AUR) is a complication of bladder outflow obstruction (BOO). It is characterised by an inability to pass urine, despite a strong desire to do so, rapid onset and lower abdominal or urethral pain with an acutely tender bladder on abdominal examination.

Clinical features

AUR may be precipitated by a high fluid intake, overdistension due to delayed voiding and reduced contractility of the bladder muscle due to overstretching. Any upper tract obstruction caused by AUR is usually rapidly relieved by bladder decompression.

The risk factors for developing AUR are shown in Table 1. As a surrogate marker of prostate volume, an elevated prostate-specific antigen (PSA) indicates a large gland with a greater risk of urinary retention (Fig. 1). The probability of a 60-year-old man

developing AUR by the time he reaches 80 is in the region of 23%.

Post-operative AUR often results from a series of events including confinement to bed, increased fluid intake from intravenous infusions, drugs that affect detrusor contractility, post-operative pain and constipation. A number of epidemiological studies have also linked urinary retention to general and spinal anaesthesia.

Management

AUR is exquisitely painful and requires immediate catheterisation. This can usually be carried out urethrally but, if any difficulties are encountered with the insertion of a urethral catheter, suprapubic catheterisation can be performed to relieve symptoms.

If the patient has a urinary tract infection (UTI) without pre-existing lower urinary tract symptoms (LUTS), gross constipation, a provocative drug

aetiology or a low (<500 mL) residual volume, a trial without catheter (TWOC) may be appropriate. All these conditions have a high probability of a successful TWOC and, in addition, delaying the TWOC to 7 days after catheterisation further increases the chance of success from 44% to 62% (Fig. 2).

In most patients, however, AUR is a complication of BOO and is best treated by surgical relief of the outflow obstruction. Surgery involves transurethral resection of the prostate (TURP), transurethral incision of the prostate (TUIP), holmium laser

Table 1 **Risk factors for the development of AUR**	
Risk factor	**Increased risk of AUR**
Age > 70 years	Eightfold
Prostate symptom score (I-PSS) > 7/35	Threefold
Prostate volume > 30 mL	Threefold
Free urinary flow rate < 12 mL/s	Fourfold
PSA > 1.4 ng/mL	Ninefold

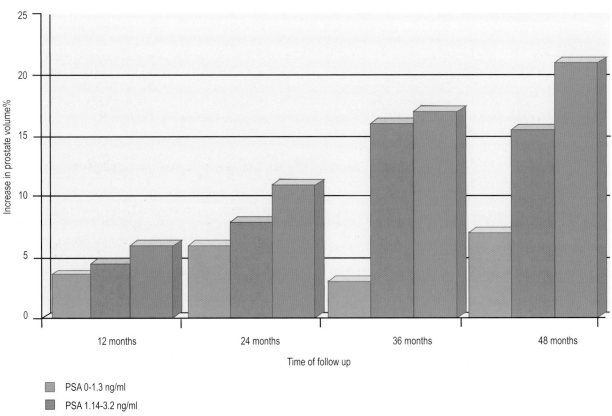

- PSA 0-1.3 ng/ml
- PSA 1.14-3.2 ng/ml
- PSA 3.2-12 ng/ml

Fig. 1 **Volume change of the prostate over time** based on serum PSA levels.

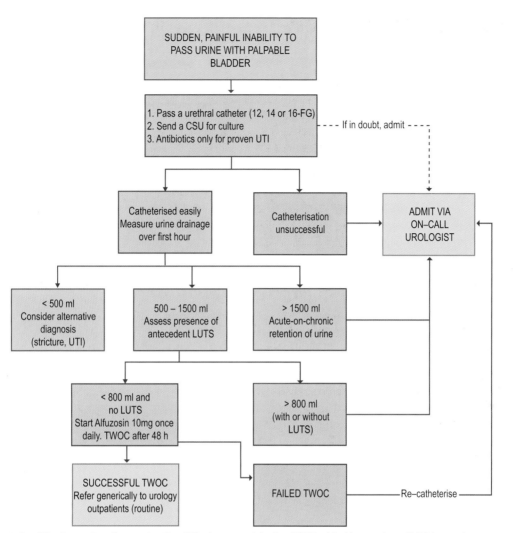

Fig. 2 **Treatment algorithm for acute urinary retention.** UTI, urinary tract infection; TWOC, trial without catheter; LUTS, lower urinary tract symptoms.

enucleation of the prostate (HOLEP) or open prostatectomy for very large glands. Surgery after acute retention has a higher morbidity, particularly from bleeding, and a threefold higher mortality (1–2%) than elective prostatectomy. Laser surgery may, however, reduce the risk of bleeding.

Approximately 20% of patients developing post-operative AUR have antecedent BOO. For those who do not have prior symptoms, a trial of voiding and institution of intermittent self-catheterisation may be preferable to immediate surgery.

Pharmacotherapy

AUR is an undesirable event for the patient. A number of studies have looked at the role of 5α-reductase inhibitors, which produce a prostate volume reduction of approximately 20% after 6 months of treatment and which may prevent AUR.

The risk of retention over 5 years is reduced by 68% in patients given a 5α-reductase inhibitor. Dual therapy with α-blockers, which reduce smooth muscle tone within the prostate and bladder neck, and 5α-reductase inhibitors has shown an even greater reduction (81%) in the risk of AUR.

Treatment of acute urinary retention

The use of α-blockers has also been explored in patients who present with their first episode of AUR. In patients given α-blockers who have no antecedent symptoms, small prostates and low PSA levels, the chance of successful voiding after catheter removal increases from 29% to 55%. However, follow-up studies have shown that more than 75% of these patients have subsequent episodes of urinary retention requiring further treatment, including surgery, over the next 5 years.

Key points

- Acute urinary retention is a complication of bladder outflow obstruction.
- Post-operative urinary retention is due to bladder outflow obstruction in approximately 20% of cases.
- The risk of acute urinary retention can be reduced by using 5α-reductase inhibitors or dual therapy with α-blockers and 5α-reductase inhibitors.
- Acute urinary retention due to bladder outflow obstruction is best treated by surgery.
- The complications of surgery are greater in patients presenting with acute urinary retention.

Chronic retention of urine

Unlike acute retention, chronic retention is painless and is defined as retention with a residual volume of >300 mL remaining in the bladder. There are two major categories, high-pressure chronic retention (HPCR) and low-pressure chronic retention (LPCR), distinguished by the bladder pressure at the end of voiding.

Table 1 **Clinical effects of high-pressure chronic retention**
Upper urinary tract dilatation (hydronephrosis)
Renal impairment
Hypertension in 50%
Congestive cardiac failure with peripheral oedema in 20%

High-pressure chronic retention (HPCR)

In HPCR, the bladder is poorly compliant, and the intravesical pressure is >25 cm of water at the end of voiding. The intravesical pressure remains consistently high, and this creates functional obstruction of the upper renal tracts with resulting chronic renal failure (Fig. 1).

Clinical features
Patients with HPCR often have few symptoms. However, nocturnal enuresis is common, and the sudden onset of this symptom in a man over the age of 50 years should raise the suspicion of HPCR. Normal transit of urine from the renal pelvis to the bladder depends on peristalsis within the ureter and the hydrostatic pressure gradient between the kidneys and the bladder. In HPCR, upper tract drainage can occur only in the erect position (due to gravity); the effects of back-pressure on the kidneys in HPCR are shown in Table 1.

Management
HPCR requires immediate decompression of the urinary tract to relieve symptoms and reduce upper tract pressures. Decompression by urethral catheterisation is the best way of achieving this, but is often followed by a post-obstructive diuresis due to the osmotic effect of high urea levels, loss of the corticomedullary concentration gradient and a net loss of sodium; it may also lead to post-decompressional haematuria. Catheterisation often allows blood pressure to return to normal and may relieve the peripheral oedema.

Following decompression, hourly urine measurements should be performed to identify any post-obstructive diuresis. Standing/lying blood pressure and daily weight are good indicators of circulating volume and fluid balance. Most patients can maintain their fluid balance by simple oral intake, but 10% require intravenous fluid replacement. Close monitoring of electrolytes and creatinine on a daily basis needs to be performed, with particular attention to sodium and potassium levels, and it is advisable to await stabilisation of renal function before attempting definitive treatment.

Patients with HPCR are best treated by prostatectomy, and outcomes are good because post-operative voiding is efficient due to preserved detrusor function. However, it is essential to monitor residual volumes and renal function post-operatively because a proportion of patients can slip back into renal failure due to recurrent obstruction without developing significant symptoms. If residual volumes are large in the post-operative period, urodynamic studies are indicated to determine whether the bladder outlet obstruction has been completely relieved. If it has, intermittent self-catheterisation may be necessary to reduce residual volumes and protect the upper tracts.

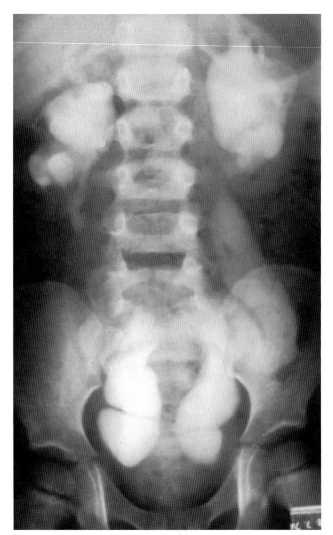

Fig. 1 High-pressure **chronic retention** in a child (the bladder is not opacified because the large residual urine has diluted the contrast medium).

Low-pressure chronic retention (LPCR)

In LPCR, the bladder is compliant and pressures remain low within the bladder during filling. Complete detrusor failure can result in huge residual volumes, and the patient may simply notice increasing girth. Lower urinary tract symptoms are often mild or non-existent, and there is no impairment of upper tract function or any of the associated cardiovascular abnormalities found in HPCR (see Fig. 2).

Most patients with LPCR require urodynamic studies before deciding on treatment because many have complete

Filling and voiding cystometry

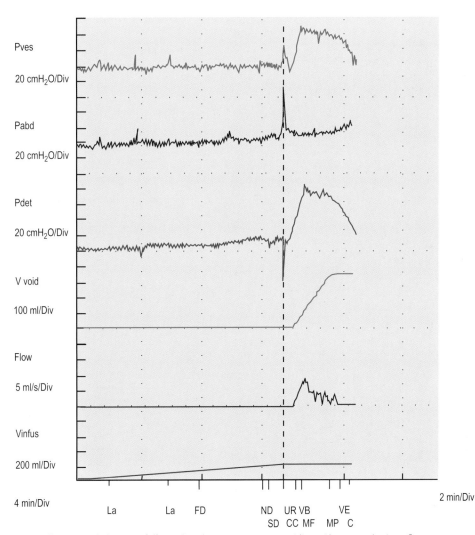

Fig. 2 Urodynamic tracing of patient with **detrusor failure** – low detrusor pressure on voiding with poor peak urinary flow rate.

detrusor failure. Although patients with LPCR may benefit from prostatectomy, large residual volumes may persist post-operatively, and intermittent self-catheterisation (ISC) may be necessary to achieve complete bladder emptying. ISC is often used as the sole treatment in complete detrusor failure, thereby avoiding the complications of surgery. Some patients with minimal symptoms, residual volumes < 500 mL and normal renal function can be managed by conservative means because they rarely progress to HPCR; such patients must, however, be monitored carefully with ultrasound and regular renal function measurements.

> *Key points*
>
> ■ Chronic retention is a complication of bladder outflow obstruction.
>
> ■ Chronic retention is divided into high-pressure (HPCR) and low-pressure (LPCR) forms dependent on the intravesical pressure at the end of voiding.
>
> ■ HPCR is associated with upper tract dilatation and renal impairment.
>
> ■ HPCR is best treated by bladder outlet surgery.
>
> ■ LPCR is best managed by urodynamics and bladder outlet surgery if there is reasonable detrusor function and intermittent self-catheterisation if detrusor function is poor.

Transurethral resection of the prostate (TURP)

TURP is indicated in patients who fail to respond to pharmacotherapy, in those who elect for surgery as a primary treatment and in those patients with complications of bladder outflow obstruction (BOO; Table 1). A Caucasian man has a lifetime risk of needing TURP in the order of 25–30%, whereas the lifetime risk in men of Asian or Oriental origin is only 10–12%.

The majority of patients requiring surgery for BOO undergo TURP, with transurethral incision of the prostate (TUIP; sometimes called bladder neck incision) being used for small-volume prostates (≤30 mL). In patients with very large prostate glands (>100–150 mL), open (retropubic or transvesical) prostatectomy may still be indicated, although laser prostatectomy is increasingly being used for very large glands. TURP, however, remains the 'gold standard' treatment for BOO, with which other treatments must be compared; the procedure has now been established for over 40 years, and good long-term follow-up data are available.

Practical considerations

TURP is performed under spinal or general anaesthetic using a continuous irrigating resectoscope of 26 French gauge (Fig. 1). The large gauge of this instrument relative to the normal urethra means that it is sometimes necessary to perform dilatation of the urethra or urethrotomy to reduce the risk of post-operative urethral stricture. The aim of treatment is to open the bladder neck and create a barrel-shaped cavity within the prostatic urethra (Fig. 2) between the bladder neck and verumontanum, the latter structure being the surgical landmark of the distal sphincter complex. The occluding prostate tissue is removed piecemeal using an electrocautery loop, and the chippings created wash forwards into the bladder from where they are then evacuated. Meticulous haemostasis is obtained, and an irrigating (three-way) urethral catheter is inserted. The catheter is removed once any haematuria has settled (usually 36–48 h after the procedure), and the average hospital stay is 4 days.

Results of TURP

At least 85% of patients undergoing TURP obtain good symptomatic relief, being satisfied with the outcome 1 year post-operatively. Symptom relief has good durability with 75% of patients still satisfied with the outcome after 3 years. Poor

Table 1 **Complications of bladder outlet obstruction (BOO)**
Acute retention
High-pressure chronic retention (HPCR)
Some men with low-pressure chronic retention (LPCR)
Renal impairment (due to chronic retention)
Recurrent urinary tract infections and/or recurrent epididymitis
Bladder calculi
Recurrent haematuria (originating from the prostate)

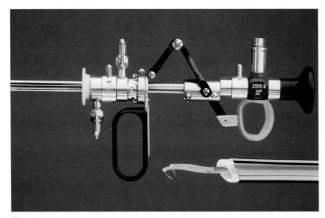

Fig. 1 **A resectoscope used to perform TURP.**

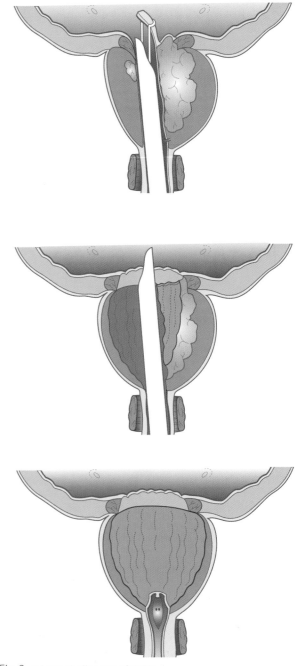

Fig. 2 **Schematic diagram of TURP.**

results are obtained when the procedure is performed in an attempt to improve storage (irritative) symptoms rather than voiding (obstructive) symptoms.

Complications

The overall morbidity of TURP ranges from 3% to 18%, but mortality rates are less than 1%, except in patients undergoing the procedure for treatment of acute retention, in whom mortality rates may be as high as 2–3%. The main complications are urinary infection (especially if the patient has had a urethral catheter prior to surgery), bleeding requiring transfusion, urethral stricture, bladder neck contracture and erectile dysfunction (Table 2). It is important that all patients are warned about the likelihood of *retrograde ejaculation*, especially those men who are sexually active.

The *TUR syndrome*, a dilutional hyponatraemia caused by absorption of large volumes of the irrigant, is a rare but significant complication. If the prostatic capsule is breached during resection and periprostatic veins are opened during the procedure, large volumes of irrigant may be absorbed into the circulation, resulting in confusion, hypertension, nausea, vomiting, visual disturbances and cardiovascular changes. This is more likely to occur with prolonged procedures, when the capsule has been perforated and when there is significant bleeding requiring high irrigation rates to allow visualisation of the operative field. The condition is managed by fluid restriction, slowing the rate of bladder irrigation and, if necessary, intravenous diuretics; hypertonic saline should not be given to correct the hyponatraemia because it is caused by fluid overload and not by a reduction in intravascular sodium levels.

Table 2 **Complications of transurethral resection of the prostate (TURP)**

Complication	Incidence
Retrograde ejaculation	90%
Impotence (erectile dysfunction)	4–40%
Urinary infection	Cystitis in 10–15%
	Epididymitis in 1%
Bleeding requiring transfusion	5–10%
Urethral stricture	5%
Bladder neck contracture	3%
Urinary incontinence	Stress incontinence in 2%
	Urge incontinence in 2%
	Total incontinence in 1%

Transurethral incision of prostate (TUIP) or bladder neck incision (BNI)

The long-term efficacy and safety of TUIP compares favourably with TURP. The procedure is shorter, there is less bleeding than in TURP, and the TUR syndrome is very rare. TUIP is indicated in patients with bladder neck hypertrophy only or in those with small-volume prostates (≤ 30 mL). It is performed using a simple 'spike' (Colling's knife), and no tissue is resected, an incision simply being made through the bladder neck to the verumontanum.

The outcomes and morbidity of TUIP are similar to those of TURP, but the risk of retrograde ejaculation may be as low as 20%, erectile dysfunction is seen in less than 10%, and blood transfusion is rarely required. Performing TURP in patients with such small prostates is contraindicated because of the risk of subsequent bladder neck contracture.

> *Key points*
>
> - TURP remains the 'gold standard' procedure to relieve bladder outlet obstruction.
> - TURP is the treatment of choice in patients with complications from bladder outlet obstruction.
> - The overall complication rate is between 3% and 18%.
> - The most significant side-effects are urinary infection, the need for blood transfusion, urethral strictures, sexual dysfunction and urinary incontinence.
> - For small-volume prostates (≤ 30 mL), TUIP produces equivalent outcomes to TURP.

Alternatives to prostatectomy

In recent years, there has been a proliferation in interventions that provide an alternative to transurethral resection of the prostate (TURP) for treatment of patients with lower urinary tract symptoms (LUTS) due to bladder outlet obstruction (BOO). The most widely used of these are shown in Table 1. Most of these techniques have been developed to reduce the morbidity of TURP and to shorten hospital stay.

Pharmacotherapy

The widespread use of pharmacotherapy as the initial treatment for LUTS has resulted in a marked reduction in the number of patients undergoing operative procedures for the relief of LUTS. Both α-adrenoceptor blockers and 5α-reductase inhibitors improve symptom scores and quality of life in men with LUTS. The former have a more rapid action, often producing improvement within 2 weeks; side-effects are seen in 10% of patients, especially nasal congestion, headache, sexual dysfunction and postural hypotension. 5α-Reductase inhibitors have a slower action but also improve urinary symptoms, especially in patients with larger prostates. Combination therapy with both of these agents reduces the risk of developing complicated BOO and reduces the risk of surgery by 50% when taken for 4 years. The low risk of side-effects and the ability to improve quality of life with these drugs makes them the treatment of first choice when managing LUTS in men with uncomplicated BOO. The balance between efficacy and side-effects of alternative treatments is shown in Fig. 1.

Alternative surgical techniques

New techniques to enucleate or destroy prostate tissue are designed to mimic TURP by producing a cavity that widens the bladder outlet. The National Institute of Health and Clinical Excellence (NICE) has evaluated a number of these techniques, and the conclusions are listed in Table 1.

Thermotherapy and cryotherapy

Applying heat to the prostate (thermotherapy) through the rectal wall or via the urethra is an attractive alternative to TURP because it is an outpatient procedure with low morbidity. The tissue effect depends on the local response to high temperatures, the nature of the prostatic tissue and prostatic vascularity. Cryotherapy is less popular but is currently being investigated in carcinoma of the prostate.

Laser techniques

Laser prostatectomy has evolved over the last 10 years to its present position as an equivalent procedure to TURP. Although time consuming, the ability to produce a resection cavity with less bleeding, a shorter hospital stay and a shorter period of catheterisation makes it likely to have a long-term role in the treatment of BOO.

HOLEP (Fig. 2) involves enucleation of the prostate and, in effect, reproduces the operation of open enucleative prostatectomy. Thermal energy, generated by a 100-W holmium laser, is transmitted along a 550-μm laser fibre passed through a 26 French gauge resectoscope using normal saline for irrigation. The three lobes of the prostate

Table 1 **Alternatives to prostatectomy**	
Intervention	**NICE approval**
Pharmacotherapy	
α-Adrenoreceptor blockers	Yes
5α-Reductase inhibitors	Yes
Combination therapy	Yes
Phytotherapy (plant extracts)	Yes
Laser technology	
HOLEP (holmium laser enucleation of the prostate)	Qualified
HOLAP (holmium laser ablation of the prostate)	Qualified
'Green light' (KTP laser) ablation	Qualified
Interstitial laser coagulation (ILC)	No
TUNA (transurethral radiofrequency needle ablation)	Qualified
Hyperthermia/cryotherapy	Qualified
HIFU (high-intensity focused ultrasound)	No
Electrovaporisation	Qualified

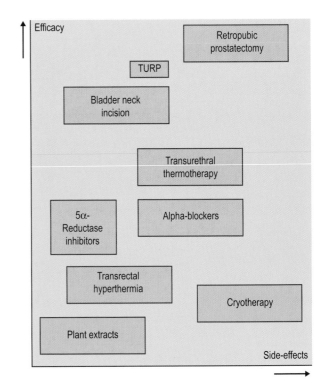

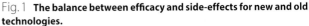

Fig. 1 **The balance between efficacy and side-effects for new and old technologies.**

(two lateral and one middle) are displaced into the bladder, where they are morcellated and extracted using a suction device with rotating blades. The main advantages of this technique are lack of bleeding and the use of saline as irrigation (thereby avoiding the *TUR syndrome*). The catheter is usually removed within 24 h of surgery, reducing hospital stay. The outcome in terms of relief of BOO and durability are equivalent to TURP at up to 4 years. To speed up the process of creating a resection cavity, potassium titanylphosphate (KTP) laser vaporisation ('green light' laser) is also gaining popularity.

Contact laser techniques vaporise tissue but are time consuming. They produce equivalent results to TURP, but retreatment rates are higher and the effects less durable.

Interstitial laser coagulation (ILC) serves to produce an area of coagulative necrosis around laser fibres inserted into the prostate via a transurethral or perineal route. The procedure causes a 20% reduction in gland volume, but is

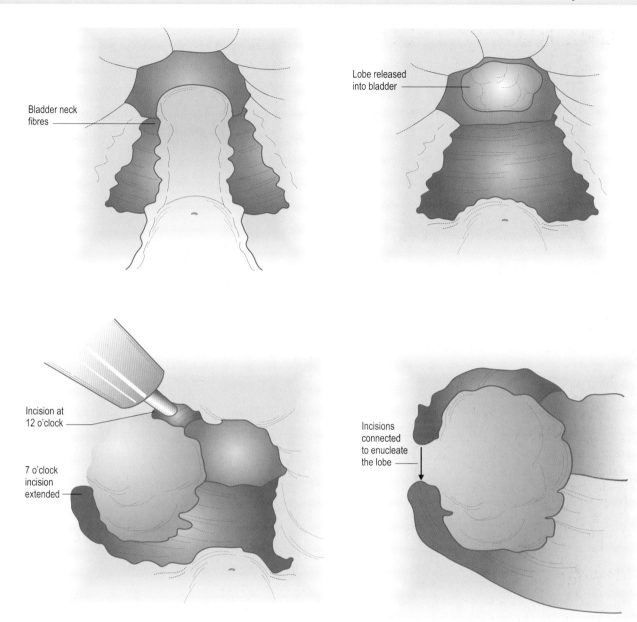

Fig. 2 **Holmium laser enucleation of the prostate** (HOLEP).

also likely to cause an alteration in neuromuscular function. Symptomatic benefit lasts for at least 3 years, but the repeat treatment rate is in the order of 16%.

Radiofrequency techniques

Transurethral needle ablation (TUNA) of the prostate involves placing needles into the prostate and applying low-level radiofrequency to create coagulative necrosis. The response to treatment improves over time with a mean improvement in prostate symptom scores of 50% at 6 months. Although the improvement in post-operative urinary flow may not be as good as that achieved after TURP, overall symptom improvement and quality of life produced are improved to a similar degree, and outlet obstruction is relieved in approximately 50%. The side-effects of urinary retention (in 13–42%), haematuria and painful voiding are the major problems of this technique. Retrograde ejaculation, erectile dysfunction, urethral strictures and incontinence are all rare, making this an acceptable procedure to patients. Its role may be for unfit patients with mild to moderate BOO and small prostates.

> ### Key points
>
> - The number of patients willing to undergo surgical procedures for their lower urinary tract symptoms (LUTS) has decreased as a result of the improved efficacy and side-effect profile of pharmacological agents (α-blockers and 5α-reductase inhibitors).
>
> - Combination therapy has the ability to reduce the complications of bladder outlet obstruction and the need for surgery by 50% when used over a 4-year period.
>
> - Thermotherapy can reduce LUTS and is associated with a low side-effect profile and ease of delivery as an outpatient procedure.
>
> - Laser prostatectomy, particularly HOLEP, is associated with less bleeding, a shorter hospital stay and shorter period of catheterisation, and is able to create a cavity in the same way as TURP.
>
> - Transurethral needle ablation (TUNA) and interstitial laser coagulation (ILC) create less tissue loss, but may produce adequate results in patients with smaller glands.
>
> - Minimally invasive techniques are acceptable to patients because of shorter hospital stay and improved side-effect profiles, but are likely to be less efficacious and durable.
>
> - Randomised controlled trials comparing these techniques with TURP are lacking.

Incontinence and Neurourology

Assessment and urodynamic studies

Most patients with urinary incontinence can be assessed simply without the need for urodynamics. A multidisciplinary approach to assessment and management is strongly preferred and, in this respect, patients often relate better to non-medical staff than doctors.

History and examination

The key features of the history are shown in Table 1. Numerous symptom scoring systems are available, which may facilitate assessment and the response to treatment. History taking may require a rather broader assessment than is traditionally done by general practitioners (GPs), including details such as prolapse, sexual function and faecal incontinence. Examination of the abdomen, prostate, urethra, introitus, vagina and neurology are essential, with particular attention to the presence of a palpable bladder, estrogenisation status, urethral abnormalities and any pelvic masses.

Investigations

The most important investigation is *simple urine testing* to exclude other diagnoses such as infection or bladder cancer; many patients referred with incontinence are found on simple testing to have a previously undetected intravesical abnormality.

A *frequency–volume chart* (see Appendix, p. 149) is helpful for both patient and clinician. It may show fewer symptoms than the history might suggest or clear evidence of, for example, bladder overactivity with frequent, small-volume voids. The total daily urine output may also show that most urine passage occurs at night, suggesting nocturnal polyuria due to poor water handling by the kidneys.

A *urinary flow rate* may be normal (Fig. 1), supranormal (suggestive of bladder overactivity) or reduced (due to bladder hypocontractility). Significant residual urine (more

than 100 mL) on a post-micturition ultrasound scan may also suggest detrusor hypocontractility.

A *pad test*, with weighing of incontinence pads over 24–72 h, is helpful in estimating the degree of urine loss. Pad tests have been shown to be an objective and reproducible means of assessing the degree of incontinence and monitoring the response to treatment.

Urodynamics

Urodynamics should be reserved for those patients who fail conservative management and who wish to consider surgical treatment. The questions that need to be answered by urodynamics are shown in Table 2.

A urodynamic tracing from a patient with bladder outlet obstruction is shown in Fig. 2; there is a high detrusor

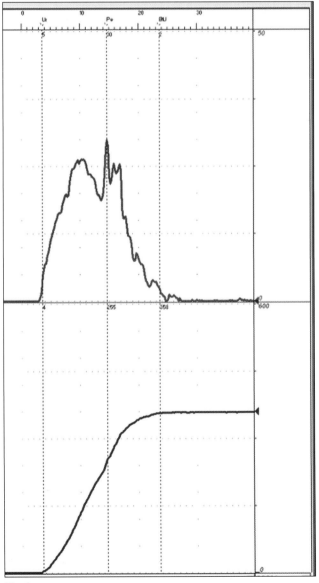

Fig. 1 **Normal urinary flow rate curve.**

Table 1 **Important factors in the history of patients with incontinence**	
Duration	A short history is suspicious of a structural bladder abnormality (stone or tumour)
Haematuria	Suspicious of bladder tumour
Degree of pad usage	Marker of the degree of incontinence
Circumstances of leakage	On standing up, 'key in the door' or handwashing (classic symptoms of bladder overactivity)
Pelvic surgical and obstetric history	Birthweights and assisted deliveries
Medication	See pp. 98 and 99
Mobility	Poor mobility may reduce 'warning time' to the point of incontinence
Pelvic prolapse	
Sexual function	
Faecal incontinence	
Frequency of symptoms	

pressure and a low voiding flow rate. Urodynamics in stress urinary incontinence (SUI) are used to confirm the leakage and to exclude associated detrusor overactivity or hypocontractility. Videourodynamics allow leakage into a pad to be seen directly without the need to inspect the patient's perineum repeatedly. Detrusor overactivity (Fig. 3) is found with conventional urodynamics in 70% of those who have it. Using a low filling rate (20 mL/min or less) improves the chances of detecting detrusor overactivity, and unstable contractions may be provoked during the study by standing, coughing or handwashing.

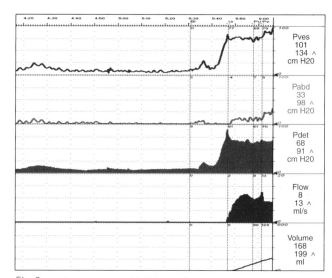

Fig. 2 Urodynamic trace in **bladder outflow obstruction** (subtracted detrusor pressure in red).

Table 2 **Urodynamic questions in urinary incontinence**		
Patient group	**Urodynamic questions to be answered**	**Clinical relevance**
Men	Presence of bladder outlet obstruction	Is bladder outlet surgery appropriate?
	Presence of detrusor hypocontractility	Will the bladder empty after bladder outlet surgery?
Women with stress urinary incontinence (SUI)	Objective evidence of SUI	Sphincter weakness?
	Stress leak point pressure	Will the bladder empty after SUI surgery?
	Presence of detrusor hypocontractility	
	Evidence of overactive detrusor	Will there be symptoms of overactive bladder after SUI surgery?
Women with overactive bladder	Evidence of overactive detrusor	
	Presence of detrusor hypocontractility	Will the bladder empty after treatment for an overactive detrusor?
	Objective evidence of SUI	Will SUI persist after intervention for an overactive detrusor?

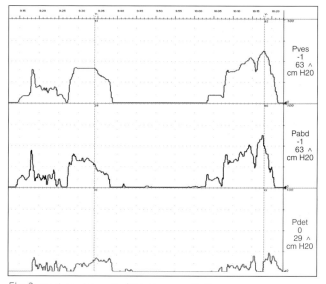

Fig. 3 Urodynamic trace in **detrusor overactivity.**

Treatment of incontinence

Conservative management, based on a clinical diagnosis alone, is usually the optimum first-line treatment. Failure to respond to one form of conservative management simply requires an alternative option to be used and, if drug side-effects are a problem, these are usually reversible on withdrawing the drug. However, if surgical treatment is indicated, urodynamic proof of the diagnosis is mandatory because symptoms are not a reliable predictor of urodynamic diagnosis.

Stress urinary incontinence (SUI)

Containment and management of fluids and voiding may be the only practical options for many frail or elderly patients unable to cooperate with more complex treatments. As a general principle, however, treatment should be directed at reducing the incontinence rather than containing it.

Pelvic floor physiotherapy
Pelvic floor physiotherapy has been shown to be very effective in controlled clinical trials, with 60% of women responding to pelvic floor exercises. Standard pelvic floor exercises are more effective than either Kegel exercises (retaining graduated weights within the vagina by pelvic floor contraction) or electrostimulation via the rectum.

Medication
The first drug licensed for use in SUI was duloxetine, to which 60% of patients respond; contrary to expectation, there is some evidence that it is effective regardless of the degree of SUI. It probably works by stimulating *Onuf's nucleus* in the sacral cord, resulting in an increase in urethral sphincter activity. The principal side-effect is nausea, which often resolves after the first month of treatment.

Surgical treatment
Surgical treatment of SUI in women is reserved for those who fail conservative treatment, but patients must be adequately counselled in advance about the possible side-effects of surgery (Table 1). Following a *suburethral sling procedure* (Fig. 1) or *colposuspension* (Fig. 2), 90% of women will be dry (or almost so), but the success rate at 10 years decreases to 60%. There are, however, no long-term follow-up data for autologous and prosthetic slings.

Periurethral injections of inert, bulking agents produce less durable effects and are usually reserved for patients who are unfit for other procedures, for the elderly and for those with low-volume leakage. Too little attention has been paid to the possible side-effects of surgery for SUI. A woman who exchanges SUI for an overactive bladder post-operatively, without being aware that this could happen, may feel badly treated.

SUI in men is most often seen after transurethral or open radical prostatectomy. If pelvic floor physiotherapy is ineffective, periurethral injections may be used but, in more severe cases, consideration should be given to insertion of an artificial urinary sphincter (AUS; Fig. 3). This carries a 90% satisfaction rate, but the revision rate is 30%, usually for complications such as mechanical failure and erosion into the urethra.

Table 1 **Side-effects of surgery for stress urinary incontinence (SUI)**	
Bladder overactivity	6–8%
Short-term voiding difficulty	5–10%
Long-term chronic retention (requiring intermittent self-catheterisation)	1–2%
Pelvic organ prolapse	33%
Tape erosion (with prosthetic suburethral slings)	3–4%

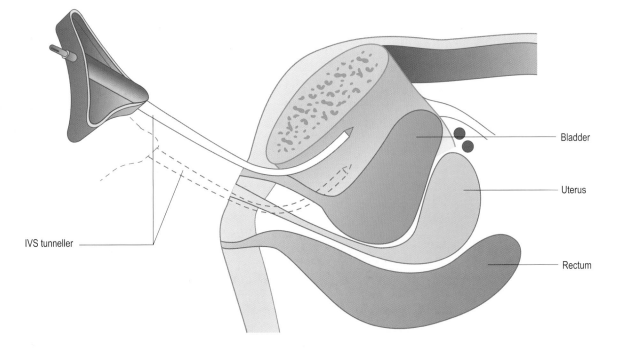

IVS tunneller

Bladder

Uterus

Rectum

Supine position

Fig. 1 **Suburethral sling procedure** (transvaginal tape, TVT).

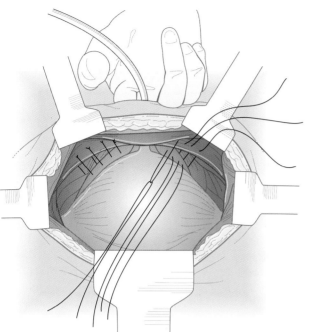

Fig. 2 **Colposuspension.**

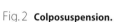

Fig. 3 **Artificial urinary sphincter** (AUS).

Overactive bladder (OAB)

The conservative options for SUI are also appropriate for OAB with the addition of *bladder training* (Table 2). When bladder training was first introduced, it involved prolonged admission to hospital for close supervision. Although this is no longer deemed appropriate, bladder training at home may still be effective in up to 85% of patients.

Medication

Most of the medications used in OAB have an anticholinergic effect, probably on M3 receptors in the detrusor. The drugs used include oxybutynin, tolterodine, propiverine, trospium and solfenacin. There is little to choose between individual agents, but slow-release preparations tend to be preferred because they have fewer side-effects. Sixty per cent of patients obtain a useful response, and there is good evidence that this is sustained over a period of time. The commonest side-effects of these drugs include dry mouth and eyes, blurred vision, dyspepsia, bowel disturbance and confusion (especially in the elderly).

Surgical treatment

For many years, surgical treatment of the overactive bladder, when conservative treatment failed, involved major surgery to augment the bladder with a bowel patch, which acted as a bladder diverticulum to 'mop up' sudden pressure rises associated with inappropriate detrusor contractions. In recent years, other techniques such as neuromodulation and intravesical injections of botulinum toxin have become popular because they are less invasive. Surgical treatment of the overactive bladder is discussed on pp. 102 and 103.

Table 2 **Bladder training for overactive bladder (OAB)**
When the desire to void occurs, try to resist the urge for 5–15 min
Do this consistently for each void over a 4- to 6-week period
Use any means of distraction to resist the urge (mental arithmetic, grit teeth, contract pelvic floor, twiddle toes)
Try to increase this 'delay' interval gradually as time goes on

NB. This treatment has no side-effects and provides durable results.

Key points

- Conservative treatment is often effective and has few side-effects.
- Standard pelvic floor exercises and drug therapy give good results in stress urinary incontinence (SUI).
- Surgical treatment is reserved for failure of conservative treatment and involves suburethral injections, a sling procedure or colposuspension.
- The side-effects of surgery for SUI are often underestimated.
- Medical treatment and bladder training are first-line measures for overactive bladder (OAB).
- Newer surgical techniques for OAB (e.g. botulinum toxin or neuromodulation) are now preferred to major bladder augmentation procedures.

Assessment and pathophysiology of neuropathic bladder disorders

Many neurological conditions can affect the lower urinary tract and, as a result, require the attention of urologists. There are often specific issues that are relevant to the management of these patients, including the presence of associated problems in other systems, whether the neurological condition is static or progressive and the patient's own views on their quality of life.

In general, the role of the urologist is to assess the urological condition(s) and then discuss with the patient what potential management options are suitable for that individual. Ultimately, this becomes an individual judgement for the patient and, as a result, two patients with the same neurological condition and the same urological problems arising from it may actually require different management. One example of this would be that some patients with spinal cord injury will choose the simplest option (a long-term suprapubic catheter) in order to avoid major surgery and more complex follow-up; others may choose bladder augmentation, a catheterisable stoma or an artificial sphincter as part of a requirement to be free of an indwelling catheter.

Urological problems in neurological conditions

The fundamental concern for any patient with a neurological condition is whether renal function is at risk because of the effects of the neurological abnormality on their urinary tract. Before the current understanding of urological problems in neurological patients was developed, premature death from renal failure was common; this was, for many years, the commonest cause of death in patients with spinal cord injury. This was largely due to a lack of understanding of the basic, underlying physiology. Patients injured in war, in mining accidents or when diving into shallow water developed high-pressure bladders after their injury. This condition was neither recognised nor managed effectively so that hydronephrosis, renal stones and, eventually, chronic renal failure led to premature death. More recently, it has been recognised that other issues such as bladder emptying, continence, urinary tract infection, erectile dysfunction and fertility are also important in these patients. Other non-urological concerns may also be relevant in patients with neuropathic bladder disorders (Table 1).

Static and progressive neurological conditions

Whether the neurological condition is static or progressive (Table 2) is of crucial importance to urological management. It also important to appreciate that some treatment options may require good eyesight as well as a degree of mental or manual dexterity (Table 3). If these faculties are subsequently affected by progression of the neurological condition, as is often the case in multiple sclerosis, not only may management need to

change, but the patient may already have undergone a procedure associated with significant morbidity with little or no benefit.

Classification of lower urinary tract function in neurological disorders

A number of classifications have been used over the years. However, the simplest method is to consider separately the effects on the bladder and the bladder outlet and to determine whether each is overactive, normal or underactive. The consequences of this classification are shown in Table 4.

An overactive sphincter may produce a condition called *detrusor–sphincter dyssynergia*, whereby the normal process of coordination between bladder contraction and bladder outlet relaxation is lost; there is intermittent contraction of the outlet during a voiding, leading to dramatic rises in

Table 1 Other issues in patients with neurological conditions

Bowel function, including faecal continence

Mobility

Skin condition in those who are wheelchair dependent

Mental function

Vision

Hand function

Table 2 Static and progressive neurological conditions

Static	Progressive
Spinal cord injury	Stroke disease
Spina bifida (meningomyelocele)	Dementia
Transverse myelitis	Multiple sclerosis
	Parkinson's disease

Table 3 Urological measures requiring mental function, manual dexterity or good vision

Procedure	Requirement from patient
Bladder augmentation	Likely to need intermittent self-catheterisation
Catheterisable stoma	Intermittent self-catheterisation
Artificial urinary sphincter	Pump activation

Table 4 Classification and consequences of lower urinary tract function in neurological disorders

Bladder	Bladder outlet		
	Overactive	Normal	Underactive
Overactive	Incontinence Chronic retention Hydronephrosis Renal impairment	Incontinence	Incontinence
Normal	Chronic retention	Normal	Incontinence
Underactive	Chronic retention	Chronic retention	Chronic retention Incontinence

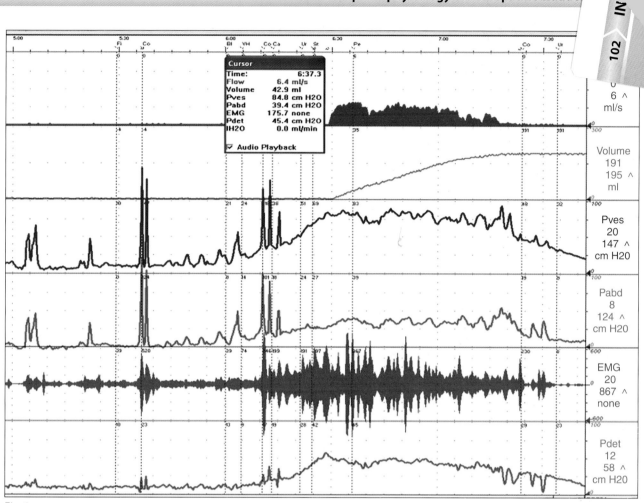

Fig. 1 Urodynamic tracing in **detrusor–sphincter dyssynergia.**

intravesical pressure. Figure 1 shows a urodynamic study in detrusor–sphincter dyssynergia, together with electromyographic (EMG) recordings from the sphincter (*sphincter EMG*); there is evidence of intermittent sphincter activity during a voiding contraction. If there are sufficient overactive bladder contractions to raise the bladder pressure to a level higher than the renal filtration pressure, upper tract dilatation develops and may progress to renal impairment. Fortunately, conditions that cause an overactive sphincter are rare, so renal impairment in neurological conditions is uncommon; it generally occurs only in spinal cord injury, spina bifida and, to a lesser extent, in Parkinson's disease. The first two conditions carry the greatest risk of upper tract deterioration.

Assessment

Assessment requires consideration of the issues in Tables 1–4. Patients with spinal cord injury or spina bifida are usually referred to urologists from a spinal injuries centre or from a paediatric urologist respectively; their management should already be in place when they are first assessed. Most other patients come from a neurologist or general practitioner. Assessment should also take into account how bladder emptying occurs (spontaneously or drained by a catheter), whether incontinence is a problem and whether urinary tract infections are occurring. The need for urodynamics is determined by whether the patient is at risk of upper tract damage and whether the current management plan is satisfactory.

Key points

- Many patient-related factors determine the management of neuropathic bladders.
- It is important to determine whether the underlying disease is static or progressive before embarking on treatment.
- The consequences of neurological disorders for the patient can be determined by assessing whether the bladder and bladder outlet are overactive, normal or underactive.
- High pressures in the bladder must be avoided because they can be transmitted to the upper tracts, resulting in renal failure and death.

Treatment of neuropathic bladder disorders

Treatment options for patients with neuropathic bladders need to be tailored to the urological problems of each individual patient. Options for management are shown in Table 1 according to the underlying urological problem; some options may need to be considered in combination.

Urinary tract infection

Repeated, symptomatic lower tract infections are best managed by *low-dose prophylactic antibiotics*. The choice of antibiotic should be determined by the risk of side-effects and the capacity for an undesirable elimination of the normal bowel flora in the long term. The optimum antibiotics in this respect are trimethoprim, cephalexin, nitrofurantoin or norfloxacin, given as a single daily dose.

Chronic retention

An *indwelling catheter* will relieve chronic retention and prevent upper tract damage if there is urodynamic evidence of a high-pressure bladder. Suprapubic catheterisation is usually preferred because changing the catheter is easy and retains dignity for the patient. Urethral catheters should be avoided in women because, in the long term, they cause erosion of the bladder neck, which causes the catheter to drop out with its balloon inflated. Permanent catheterisation is inevitably associated with chronic bacteriuria, but this does not require antibiotic treatment unless it causes systemic symptoms. Regular bladder washouts with citrate solutions may prevent long-term problems such as catheter blockage and bladder stone formation.

Intermittent self-catheterisation (ISC) is preferable if the patient has good eyesight and manual dexterity. Hydrophilic catheters are easy for the patient to insert, and the frequency of catheterisation is determined by measuring residual urine throughout the day. ISC does not run the risk of introducing infection, but actually reduces infections by removing any residual urine after voiding.

Overactive bladder (OAB)

The aim of treatment for OAB should be to reduce the pressure within the bladder, thereby protecting the upper tracts. Denervation of the bladder by *subtrigonal phenol injections* or by *endoscopic/open transection of the bladder* is no longer used because the effect is short-lived. Catheterisation or ISC should be the first measure in order to protect the kidneys.

More permanent effects can be achieved by *bladder augmentation* with an isolated patch of bowel (Fig. 1); ileum is most commonly used (*clam ileocystoplasty*). This effectively creates a large diverticulum in the vault of the bladder, which absorbs pressure rises and prevents their transmission to the upper tracts. The long-term sequelae of this procedure can be troublesome (Table 2).

Alternative treatments include dorsal rhizotomy, where the dorsal sacral roots are divided surgically to disrupt the micturition reflex arc, and implantation of a sacral root stimulator, which produces detrusor contractions and stimulates voiding. Patients undergoing dorsal rhizotomy usually require ISC after the procedure to allow bladder emptying.

Intravesical botulinum toxin is currently the preferred option for OAB due to neurological disease. The toxin is

Table 1 **Management options in neurological conditions**	
Clinical problem	**Treatment options**
Urinary tract infection	Treat chronic retention
	Consider low-dose prophylactic antibiotics
Chronic retention	Intermittent self-catheterisation
	Indwelling suprapubic catheter
	Indwelling urethral catheter
Overactive bladder	Conservative measures
	Intravesical botulinum toxin
	Neuromodulation
	Bladder augmentation
	Ileal conduit urinary diversion
	Dorsal root rhizotomy
	Sacral nerve root stimulation
Sphincter weakness (stress urinary incontinence)	Condom catheter drainage
	Indwelling catheter
	Artificial urinary sphincter
	Bladder neck closure and catheterisable stoma (*Mitrofanoff procedure*)
	Intermittent self-catheterisation
Detrusor–sphincter dyssynergia	Indwelling suprapubic catheter
	External sphincterotomy and condom drainage device
	Sphincterotomy and artificial urinary sphincter (AUS)

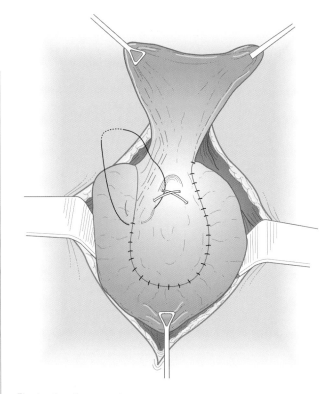

Fig. 1 **Clam ileocystoplasty.**

Table 2 **Long-term sequelae of bladder augmentation**	
Symptom	**Mechanism**
Poor bladder emptying	Reduction in bladder pressure may not allow normal voiding and intermittent self-catheterisation may be required
Mucus in the urine	Mucus plugs from the bowel may obstruct voiding Mucolytic agents may help in management
Urinary tract infection	May need low-dose prophylactic antibiotics
Bowel disturbance	Loss of reabsorption of bile salts from the terminal ileum
Metabolic abnormalities	Hyperchloraemic acidosis (due to solute absorption across the bowel patch) Osteomalacia
Malignancy	Adenocarcinoma may develop at the junction between bladder and bowel (possibly due to endogenous nitrosamines)

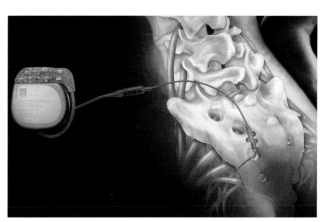

Fig. 2 **Sacral neuromodulation.**

injected into the bladder wall under local anaesthetic through a flexible cystoscope. Symptoms are relieved in 60–70% of patients, but this improvement may last only a few months; long-term follow-up data are not available.

Sacral root neuromodulation is used in some centres for OAB (Fig. 2). Following confirmation that the patient's symptoms respond to stimulation of the S3 motor root (using a temporary electrode inserted under local anaesthetic), a programmable stimulator is implanted in a subcutaneous pocket above the buttock, and the S3 root is stimulated continuously. Sixty per cent of patients with OAB refractory to other treatments respond to neuromodulation.

Urinary diversion, usually into an ileal conduit, may be necessary for some patients whose symptoms are refractory to other treatment or who want a 'one-off' solution to their problem.

Sphincter weakness

A simple *condom drainage device* or *indwelling catheter* may be appropriate for many patients, and insertion of an *artificial*

urinary sphincter (AUS), while a major procedure, produces good functional results provided the patient has adequate manual dexterity to activate the device.

One surgical alternative is to close off the neck of the bladder through a suprapubic incision and construct a catheterisable stoma on the abdomen. This involves fashioning a conduit between the bladder and the anterior abdominal wall using a flap of bladder, the appendix, a fallopian tube or an isolated segment of bowel (*Mitrofanoff procedure*). The stoma is catheterised regularly to empty the bladder.

Detrusor–sphincter dysssynergia

Division of the external sphincter (*external sphincterotomy*) is occasionally used to prevent high bladder pressures. This inevitably causes incontinence, but the incontinence can be managed either with a condom drainage device or, if the patient prefers, by implantation of an artificial urinary sphincter.

Key points

- High bladder pressures should be treated initially by an indwelling catheter or by intermittent self-catheterisation (ISC).

- Long-term reduction in bladder pressure can be accomplished by bladder augmentation with a bowel segment, dorsal rhizotomy or an anterior sacral root stimulator.

- Botulinum toxin injected into the detrusor muscle is likely to become the treatment of first choice for many patients with OAB due to neurological disease.

- Major surgery should be reserved for those patients whose symptoms are refractory to simpler measures and with whom a detailed discussion about risks and benefits has taken place.

Incontinence in the elderly

Urinary incontinence in the elderly deserves separate attention because of its prevalence, its impact on the patient, the need to involve carers and the costs to society. There are a number of issues that apply specifically to the management of incontinence in the elderly.

Categorisation of elderly patients

A distinction must be made between the elderly who are in good health, those with a particular disability (e.g. a previous stroke) and the so-called frail elderly; the last group is not easily defined but is readily recognised by clinicians. In general, the issues surrounding incontinence problems are more important in the frail elderly than in the other two groups. The ageing population is steadily increasing in number, and the prevalence of urinary

incontinence rises with age; at 60 years, approximately 20% of men and 40% of women report some degree of incontinence. The prevalence also increases markedly with increasing social dependency (Fig. 1). Patients in residential and nursing homes commonly have urinary incontinence and often have poor access to basic urological assessment and care.

Age-related factors affecting lower urinary tract function

In the elderly, a number of changes in the lower urinary tract may predispose to the development of incontinence (Table 1). These may coexist with each other and with other comorbid factors outside the lower urinary tract, resulting in loss of continence. Awareness of all these factors may allow them to be addressed in an effective manner.

There are also a number of factors outside the lower urinary tract that may lead to incontinence. Delirium is a term that should not be confused with dementia; it is associated with a variety of predisposing factors, especially urinary tract infection (common in the elderly). It typically develops over 7–10 days and may result in short-term incontinence, which resolves with effective treatment of the underlying

Table 1 **Age-related changes in the lower urinary tract**
Reduction in motor innervation of the bladder and urethra
Reduction in detrusor contractility
Reduced functional bladder capacity
Increased urinary frequency
Reduced sensation of bladder filling
Increase in prevalence of detrusor overactivity
Bladder outlet obstruction in men is more common
Estrogen-related urogenital atrophy is more common in women

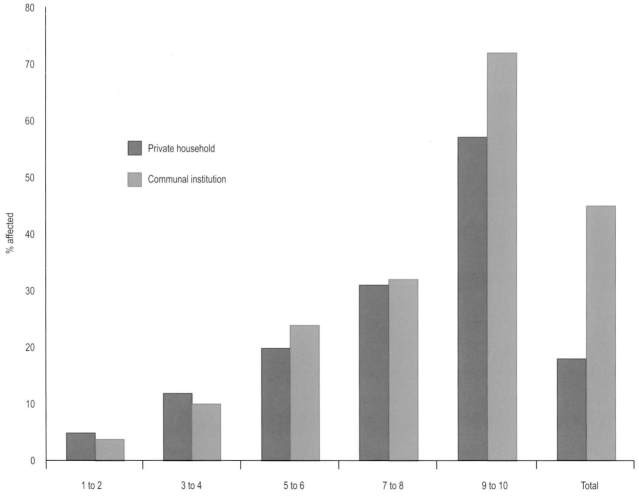

Fig. 1 Prevalence of **incontinence in elderly patients** related to the level of dependency.

cause. Urinary tract infection can produce sufficient local disturbance to lower urinary tract control (especially urgency) that continence is lost. Urogenital atrophy due to poor estrogenisation of the introitus occurs in up to 80% of elderly women, and psychological problems are common in the elderly, often related to social isolation. Concomitant drug treatment of other conditions may be important and can usually be identified from the history alone. Drinking habits may be excessive or rigid in elderly patients, and conditions such as nocturnal polyuria or diabetes insipidus may impair continence. When mobility is impaired, by either musculoskeletal disease or poor cognitive function, it may become difficult for the patient to negotiate stairs or other obstructions, and it may not be possible for the patient to delay voiding. As in many other patient groups, the interaction between lower urinary tract function and bowel function plays an important role; constipation and faecal loading are frequently linked to urinary incontinence.

The role of prescribed medications

The elderly patient is often receiving treatment for multiple conditions with a number of different medications, and physicians who care for the elderly are familiar with the problems that this can cause. Interactions between medications are more likely, and age-related changes in renal and hepatic function alter the metabolism of drugs, leading to increased toxicity with a greater likelihood of interaction.

Anticholinergic side-effects are common with many medications (Table 2), and these can interfere with normal voiding. Other drugs may contribute to incontinence because of other side-effects on the urinary tract

(Table 3). Elderly patients often fail to adhere to medication regimes, especially when large numbers of different drugs have been prescribed.

Assessment

The importance of a general assessment of the elderly patient with incontinence is underlined by the role that factors not related to the lower urinary tract play. Issues specific to the assessment of elderly patients are shown in Table 4. Particular emphasis should be placed on a thorough review of prescribed medications with attention also to the factors mentioned above.

Management

As with other patient groups, the majority of elderly patients with incontinence can be managed conservatively along standard lines with good results. The input of carers for the disabled and frail elderly is, however, very important. Treatment may involve the use of behavioural management strategies such as fluid intake management, prompted voiding and timed voiding. Such measures are time intensive and impose a significant burden on carers, and it can be difficult to sustain the benefit in institutional residents. In many patients, containment with pads or incontinence pants may be the only realistic measure. Although long-term catheterisation should be regarded as a last resort, it may be a suitable option for some patients.

Caution is needed when prescribing some medications to control the lower urinary tract; in particular, α-blockers

(postural hypotension) and anticholinergics (cognitive side-effects) may have unwanted side-effects. Nocturnal polyuria may respond to a dose of diuretic in the afternoon or to an afternoon nap (to allow fluid to return to the intravascular space). Synthetic antidiuretic hormone (ADH; desmopressin) has a role in some patients, but serum sodium levels should be monitored carefully especially when treatment is first commenced.

Surgical treatment may be indicated despite the age of the patient. Procedures such as transurethral resection of the prostate (TURP) and surgery for stress urinary incontinence can be considered on their merits when conservative measures fail and a correctable cause of incontinence has been demonstrated. However, because age-related changes in the lower urinary tract include an increased prevalence of bladder overactivity and detrusor hypocontractility, assessment before any surgery should probably include urodynamics to confirm the clinical diagnosis and minimise inappropriate intervention.

Table 4 **Additional factors in the assessment of the elderly incontinent patient**	
History	Information from carers
	Mental state assessment
	Drug history
	Mobility
	Cardiovascular symptoms
	Bowel history
Examination	Cardiovascular system
	Rectal examination
	Mental state assessment
	Estrogen status of the urogenital tissues
Investigations	Fluid intake and output (frequency–volume chart)
	Renal function

Table 3 **Drug side-effects contributing to urinary incontinence in the elderly**	
α-Blockers	Low urethral resistance
Opiates	Constipation
Anticonvulsants	Confusion
	Ataxia
Antihypertensives	Postural hypotension
Antiparkinsonian agents	Confusion
	Postural hypotension
H2-receptor blockers	Confusion
Loop diuretics	Frequency
	Urgency
Hypnotics	Excessive sedation
Minor tranquillisers	Excessive sedation
Calcium channel antagonists	Constipation
	Acute retention of urine
	Nocturnal polyuria
Angiotensin-converting enzyme inhibitors	Stress incontinence (due to coughing)

Table 2 **Drugs with anticholinergic side-effects in the elderly**	
Type of drug	**Other side-effects**
Antipsychotics	Dry mouth
Tricyclics	Constipation
Antiparkinsonian agents	Confusion
Sedating antihistamines	Drowsiness, fatigue
Disopyramide	Tachycardia
Antispasmodics	Detrusor inhibition
Opiates	Retention of urine
	Blurred vision
	Raised ocular pressure

Key points

- Incontinence increases in prevalence with increasing age.

- Age-related changes have an important bearing on the function of the lower urinary tract in the elderly.

- Prescribed medications often have side-effects that affect lower urinary tract function.

- A careful assessment should involve carers, patient and clinician.

- Management is along the usual lines, but careful urodynamic assessment is essential before any surgical intervention.

Tumours of the Genitourinary Tract

Carcinogenesis in the urinary tract

Whatever the cause of cancer, its development is a multistage process involving damage to the genes that control normal cell growth and cell division; several mutations are needed for cancer to develop. Carcinogens are either genotoxins, which cause irreversible genetic mutations (exogenous chemicals, radiation, ultraviolet light, viruses), or non-genotoxins (hormones, organic compounds), which promote cell growth.

The normal cell cycle

In the normal cell cycle (Fig. 1), an orderly progression occurs with checkpoints where DNA repair can take place; the important checkpoints are found at the G1S and G2M interfaces. The critical regulator at the G1S checkpoint is the transcription factor p53; 50% of tumours have a mutation of the *p53* gene, resulting in loss of the normal suppressor effect on DNA replication. If control is lost at the G2M checkpoint, inappropriate cell division occurs, and programmed cell death (apoptosis) is inhibited.

Exogenous carcinogens, radiation, free radicals and replication errors may result, singly or in combination, in DNA damage. If this damage can be repaired at the cell cycle checkpoints, normal growth continues. If repair is incomplete, apoptosis is normally triggered, but further gene mutations may then allow cells to bypass this process and progress to malignant transformation.

Oncogenes, including those stimulated by viruses, and a lack of tumour suppressor genes inhibit DNA repair mechanisms, allow further genetic mutations and thus permit cells to bypass the usual cycle of apoptosis, which acts to destroy genetically damaged cells. Loss of these repair mechanisms is critical to the development of cancer. Cancer cells that are protected from apoptosis by their genetic make-up have a distinct survival advantage.

Cell surface receptors (such as those for tyrosine kinase) and promoters of intercellular adhesion (E-cadherin, integrin) may also be involved in the development of cancer. Cancer cells lose their normal cell adhesion properties, and many tumour growth factors appear to act through tyrosine kinase receptors on the cell surface.

Renal cancer

Fifty per cent of patients with von Hippel–Lindau (VHL) disease develop renal cancer in middle age. Studies in both patients with VHL and those with sporadic renal carcinoma have shown this to be due to a defect in a VHL suppressor gene at chromosome 3p25–26; both alleles of the gene must mutate or be inactivated for renal cancer to develop. This genetic defect leads to overexpression of hypoxia-inducible factor I with upregulation of vascular endothelial growth factor (VEGF), resulting in angiogenesis and the new vessel formation often seen in renal cancer. There seems to be only limited involvement of oncogenes and p53 suppression in renal cancer.

Urothelial cancer

Oncogenes of the *ras* gene family (*p21 ras*) have been found in up to 50% of patients with bladder cancer. Several tumour suppressor genes have also been implicated in bladder cancer, including *p53*, retinoblastoma gene (*pRb*) and genes on the 13q, 9p21 and 9q32–33 chromosomes. *p53* directs genetically abnormal cells towards apoptosis, but mutations render the genome unstable resulting in further mutations. *p53* abnormalities are associated with more aggressive bladder cancers. Inactivation of *pRb* permits cells to go through the G1S checkpoint without DNA repair and to proliferate more easily. Amplification of genes that code for receptors of epidermal growth factor (EGF) induces cancer cell growth. Exogenous carcinogens, especially 4-aminobiphenyl, and smoking play an important role in bladder cancer; detoxification of the carcinogens responsible is usually by acetylation, and slow acetylators are known to be more prone to develop bladder cancer.

Prostate cancer

Hereditary prostate cancer is associated with a genetic defect on chromosome 1q24–25, whereas a chromosome 8p defect is seen in sporadic tumours; both these genetic defects interfere with normal tumour suppressor genes. Most prostate cancers express telomerase which, in effect, immortalises cells and leads to the production of EGF, transforming growth factor-β (TGF-β), insulin-like growth factor (IGF) and endothelin-1. Free radicals are normally inactivated by protective enzymes, and expression of these enzymes is absent in virtually all cases of prostate cancer and prostatic intraepithelial neoplasia (PIN). Oncogenes and suppressor genes (especially *p27*) are thought to play a part in the development of prostate cancer (Fig. 2) as well as in its progression and metastatic potential. Metalloproteinases may regulate the progression of PIN to invasive disease, and reduced E-cadherin expression may result in poor intercellular adhesion.

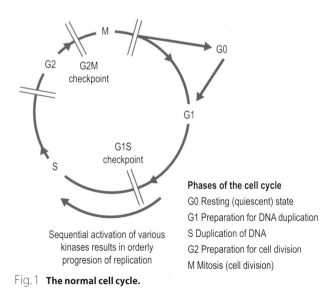

Phases of the cell cycle
G0 Resting (quiescent) state
G1 Preparation for DNA duplication
S Duplication of DNA
G2 Preparation for cell division
M Mitosis (cell division)

Sequential activation of various kinases results in orderly progresion of replication

Fig. 1 **The normal cell cycle.**

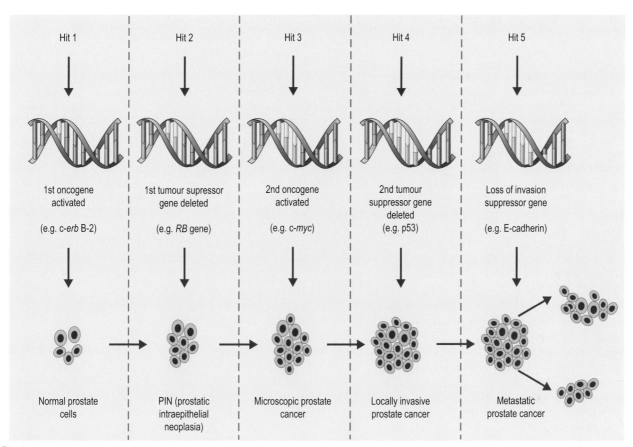

Hit 1	Hit 2	Hit 3	Hit 4	Hit 5
1st oncogene activated	1st tumour supressor gene deleted	2nd oncogene activated	2nd tumour suppressor gene deleted	Loss of invasion suppressor gene
(e.g. c-erb B-2)	(e.g. RB gene)	(e.g. c-myc)	(e.g. p53)	(e.g. E-cadherin)
Normal prostate cells	PIN (prostatic intraepithelial neoplasia)	Microscopic prostate cancer	Locally invasive prostate cancer	Metastatic prostate cancer

Fig. 2 **Oncogenes and prostate cancer.**

Testicular cancer

Congenital factors are important in the development of testicular cancer. The risk of testicular cancer in cryptorchid patients is 3–14 times normal, and 5–10% of cryptorchid patients develop tumours in the contralateral, normal testis. The timing of damage to embryonic germ cells seems to determine the potential for malignant transformation and the latent period before cancer develops.

Penile cancer

Men who have been circumcised in childhood are protected against penile cancer; the presence of a foreskin, especially in childhood, may allow unknown carcinogens to accumulate in retained smegma. Late circumcision (in adult life) conveys little protection against penile cancer. The presence of human papillomavirus (HPV) in the foreskin correlates directly with the number of sexual partners and the risk of penile cancer. Specific DNA sequences from different HPV types (16, 18, 31 and 33) are found in diseased foreskins, both benign and malignant, but not in normal foreskins. However, only 30–60% of patients with penile cancer have HPV, so additional factors must be involved. There is some evidence that tobacco products may augment the effect of HPV and chronic inflammation to promote malignant transformation.

Key points

- Malignant transformation requires multiple genetic mutations for tumour cells to develop.
- The basic underlying action of all carcinogenic agents is to inhibit the repair of abnormal or damaged DNA.
- The presence of oncogenes and downregulation of tumour suppression factors results in cells bypassing the usual process of apoptosis to become malignant.
- Many other factors then contribute to the capacity for cancer cells to progress and metastasise.
- Most urological cancers have been shown to have defects at some point in these DNA repair mechanisms.

Haematuria

The assessment of haematuria involves conditions that fall within the domain of both urologists and nephrologists. Assessment can be complicated because haematuria often presents to other clinicians who may not be fully aware of its significance and, as a result, may not investigate it appropriately. It is still not clear how we should actually define significant haematuria or how best to assess different groups of patients according to their risk. Haematuria is usually identified when patients see visible blood in their urine (*macroscopic*), when red blood cells (RBCs) are found by urine dipstick testing (*dipstick*) or when they are found on urine microscopy (*microscopic*).

Detection of blood in the urine

Macroscopic haematuria is obvious to patients and leads them to seek medical advice, often on an urgent basis; it is usually associated with other urinary symptoms (especially those of infection), but painless haematuria is the hallmark of urothelial malignancy. Microscopic haematuria is usually detected during assessment for other conditions and is often ignored by clinicians on the basis that, if it is not macroscopic, it is not significant. Delaying assessment for repeated testing of the urine is probably inappropriate, but retesting is positive in only 65% of patients, and red cells are confirmed in the urine on microscopy in only 55%; persistent positive dipstick testing is seen in 16% of patients regularly retested over a 5-year period.

The dipstick test is based on a reaction between haemoglobin or myoglobin and an indicator compound, ortho-toluidine; the actual number of red cells detected on stick testing is close to the normal level of red cells in urine (Table 1). However, there is little overlap between normal and abnormal excretion of RBCs, so the dipstick test is a very useful discriminator. Free haemoglobin is found in the urine in intravascular haemolysis and rhabdomyolysis, while myoglobin is found in myoglobinuria; both haemoglobin and myoglobin can produce false-positive results. False-negative tests can be caused by high urine specific gravity, high urine pH or by consumption of large quantities of vitamin C. The correlation between dipstick findings and urine microscopy is shown in Table 2. Urine microscopy correlates poorly with dipstick findings unless the urine presented to the laboratory for examination is fresh and is examined immediately after voiding.

Prevalence

The prevalence of dipstick haematuria in adults is 3–18% over the age of 50 years and 9–13% over the age of 70 years. Young males have a 5% prevalence and children 0.1–4%. In children, microscopic haematuria is rarely due to urological disease, and nephrological advice should be sought. In adults aged less than 45 years, 30% of patients with dipstick haematuria are subsequently found to have an underlying abnormality, which is 'significant' in only 2%; there are no malignancies in most reported series. Long-term follow-up of these patients shows that the urine dipstick remains positive over the next 7 years.

In adults over 45 years, and in those at high risk of urothelial cancer due to smoking, an underlying abnormality will be identified in 55–80%, but this is deemed 'significant' in only 20%; of these, half will be malignant, giving an overall 10% risk of malignancy in this group. With macroscopic haematuria, 35% of patients have a 'significant' abnormality, and the overall risk of malignancy is in the order of 15–20%.

Classification

It is possible, in some patients, to determine the site of bleeding in the urinary tract, and this can help to determine the most appropriate investigations. The presence of red cell casts on urine microscopy is indicative of a renal cause, but it can be difficult to determine the actual site of blood loss. Phase contrast microscopy has been used to distinguish between glomerular haematuria (where the RBCs are dysmorphic) and lower tract bleeding (where the cells are eumorphic). If > 90% of the RBCs are dysmorphic, this is indicative of a renal parenchymal abnormality but, if the pattern is mixed or > 90% of RBCs are eumorphic, it is likely that the cause lies in the lower urinary tract, and full urological assessment is needed.

Causes

The commonest causes of haematuria are shown in Table 3. The age of presentation strongly influences the likely cause of bleeding, as does the presence of proteinuria or hypertension, which usually indicate a nephrological abnormality.

In general, all patients with macroscopic haematuria should be assessed to determine the cause of their bleeding. When dipstick haematuria is found, high-risk patients (over 45 years, smokers) should be fully investigated. There is, however, a tendency for urologists to neglect nephrological causes and subject too many patients to cystoscopy.

Failure to detect previously undiagnosed platelet disorders or coagulopathy may lead to major haemorrhagic complications during subsequent investigations or after

---

Table 1 Quantification of blood in the urine

A normal patient loses 40 000 red blood cells (RBCs)/h in the urine

Normal red cell excretion in the urine is 3500 RBCs/mL (1 or 2 RBCs per high-powered field)

5% of the normal population have > 20 000 RBCs/mL (> 8 RBCs per high-powered field) – this is termed *leaky membrane disease* or *benign familial haematuria*

The threshold for dipstick positivity is 50 000 RBCs/mL

Up to 16% of the normal population may be dipstick positive

Table 2 Correlation between dipstick findings and urine microscopy in 1000 patients

	Microscopy positive	Microscopy negative
Dipstick positive	185 (18.5%)	98 (9.8%)
Dipstick negative	300 (3.0%)	687 (68.7%)

Positive predictive value, 65%; negative predictive value, 96%; accuracy, 87%.

Table 3 **Common causes of haematuria**	
Abnormal haemostasis	Aspirin
	Clopidogrel
	Warfarin
	Heparin
	Platelet disease
	Coagulopathy
Spurious	Beetroot and other foodstuffs
	Drugs
	Flutamide
	Phenolphthalein
	Phenothiazines
	Rifampicin
	Nitrofurantoin
	Pyridium
	Haemoglobin/myoglobin
	Vegetable dyes
	High urinary urate levels
	Urine hypotonicity
	High urine pH
	Factitious (self-induced)
	'Joggers' haematuria
	Serratia marcescens urinary infection
Urological	Infection
	Pyelonephritis
	Cystitis
	Schistosomiasis (bilharzia)
	Benign prostatic hyperplasia
	Urological cancer
	Transitional cell carcinomas
	Renal tumours
	Prostate tumours
	Urinary tract calculi
	Trauma
	Papillary necrosis
	Radiation cystitis
	Arteriovenous malformations
Nephrological	IgA nephropathy
	Minimal change nephropathy
	Membranous nephropathy
	Glomerulonephritis
	Vasculitis (e.g. systemic lupus erythematosus)

surgical treatment. When patients are taking drugs that affect haemostasis, the likelihood of finding an underlying abnormality is the same as in patients taking no drugs. Haematuria per se should never be ascribed to aspirin, clopidogrel, heparin or warfarin without further investigation. For similar reasons, patients with known haematological disorders or coagulopathy should also be investigated fully.

Key points

■ Blood in the urine may be macroscopic, microscopic or dipstick detected.

■ Dipstick testing is highly accurate but correlates poorly with urine microscopy findings.

■ Studies of red cell morphology may help to localise the source of bleeding.

■ The age and risk factors of the patient usually determine the chances of detecting a significant underlying abnormality.

Renal tumours – presentation and diagnosis

Benign tumours

There are two significant benign tumours, oncocytoma and angiomyolipoma. Oncocytoma is indistinguishable from renal cell carcinoma except on histology. Angiomyolipomas (Fig. 1) are asymptomatic when small but have an increased risk of bleeding when > 4 cm. They are associated with tuberous sclerosis, mental retardation, epilepsy and adenoma sebaceum.

Malignant tumours

Renal cell carcinoma (Table 1) accounts for 2% of adult cancers with a mean age at diagnosis of 70 years and a 56% tumour-specific mortality. Increased use of abdominal imaging accounts for a greater proportion (30–60%) of tumours being diagnosed incidentally. Thirty per cent of patients have evidence of metastases at presentation.

Ninety-six per cent of renal tumours are sporadic in nature whereas 4% are inherited. The commonest inherited form is von Hippel–Lindau disease, an autosomal dominant familial cancer with mutation in the short arm of chromosome 3. The syndrome comprises renal cell carcinoma, retinal angiomas, cerebellar haemangioblastomas, phaeochromocytomas, cysts of the kidney, pancreas or epididymis, pancreatic islet cell tumours and endolymphatic sac tumours. More than 70% of patients develop renal tumours by the age of 60 years, and these are often multifocal.

There are no clear risk factors for the sporadic forms. However, smoking, obesity (in females), endstage renal disease, polycystic kidneys and hypertension are all thought to contribute.

Staging

The tumour/node/metastasis (TNM) classification of renal tumours is shown in Table 2. At diagnosis, 25–30% have metastases to lung, soft tissues, bone, liver, skin and brain in order of frequency.

Presenting features

The classic triad of loin pain, haematuria and flank mass occurs in only 10% of patients. Incidental detection of renal tumours has become commonest (30–60%). Patients may present with haematuria alone, and *paraneoplastic syndromes* are common (Table 3). Symptomatic patients are more likely to have high-grade disease.

There are often no abnormal findings on examination other than evidence of weight loss, cachexia or anaemia. Abdominal examination may reveal a palpable mass in the upper abdomen or flank. A left-sided varicocele may be seen in men with left-sided renal tumours. Lower limb oedema, suggesting nodal disease or obstruction of the inferior vena cava, is occasionally seen.

Table 1 Histological types of renal cell carcinoma

Histology	%	Cytopathology
Clear cell	80	Granular cells with abundant eosinic cytoplasm (Fig. 2)
Papillary	15	Nuclear anaplasia with granular eosinic cytoplasm
Chromophobe	4	Transparent cytoplasm
Sarcomatoid	1	Spindle cells with pleomorphic nuclei

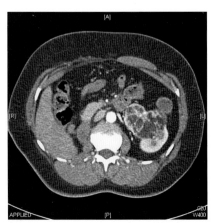

Fig. 2 **Histology of clear cell renal carcinoma.**

Table 3 Paraneoplastic syndromes associated with renal cell carcinoma

Abnormality	Frequency
Elevated erythrocyte sedimentation rate (ESR)	55%
Hypertension	35%
Anaemia	35%
Weight loss	35%
Pyrexia	15%
Stauffer syndrome	15%
Hypercalcaemia	10%
Polycythaemia	3%
Neuromyopathy	3%

Table 2 TNM staging of renal tumours

Primary tumour (T)	
TX	Primary tumour cannot be assessed
T0	No evidence of primary tumour
T1a	Tumour ≤ 4 cm limited to kidney
T1b	Tumour > 4 cm and ≤ 7 cm limited to kidney
T2	Tumour > 7 cm limited to the kidney
T3	Tumour extends into major veins or invades ipsilateral adrenal gland or perinephric tissue, but does not extend beyond Gerota's fascia
T3a	Tumour invades ipsilateral adrenal gland and perinephric fat
T3b	Tumour extends into renal vein or vena cava below diaphragm
T3c	Tumour grossly extends into renal veins and vena cava above diaphragm
T4	Tumour extends beyond Gerota's fascia and/or directly invades local strictures
Regional lymph nodes (N)	
NX	Regional lymph nodes cannot be assessed
N0	No regional lymph nodes
N1	Single ipsilateral node
N2	Metastases in more than a single regional lymph node
Metastases (M)	
MX	Distant metastases cannot be assessed
M0	No distant metastases
M1	Distant metastases

Fig. 1 CT showing an **angiomyolipoma** in the left kidney with high fat content.

Investigations

Routine investigations should include urinalysis, full blood count, erythrocyte sedimentation rate (ESR), electrolytes, creatinine and liver function tests (alkaline phosphatase and serum calcium).

Computerised tomography (CT) or ultrasound are now the first-line investigations in patients who present with frank haematuria. The former provides good anatomical detail, information about nodal status and functional information about both kidneys (Figs 3 and 4); reconstructed images can be produced if nephron-sparing treatment is to be considered. A chest radiograph is essential, and CT of the chest is performed for all suspected renal tumours > 3 cm. Bone scintigraphy to identify metastases is performed only in those patients with bone pain or an elevated alkaline phosphatase. Occasionally, ultrasound or CT-guided needle biopsy of the lesion may be necessary if there is genuine doubt about the nature of a renal mass. In patients with renal impairment, renography or measurement of glomerular filtration rate (GFR) may be necessary.

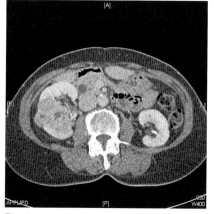

Fig. 3 CT scan with **intravenous contrast medium** showing a confined right renal carcinoma and function in both kidneys.

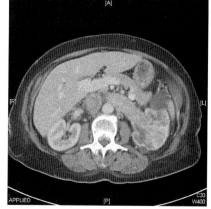

Fig. 4 **CT scan showing left renal tumour** with involvement of the left renal vein and inferior vena cava.

Key points

■ The incidence of renal cell carcinoma is increasing, and the ratio of mortality to incidence is 56%.

■ An increasing proportion of renal tumours are diagnosed incidentally (40–60%).

■ Thirty per cent of patients have metastases at presentation.

■ Ultrasound and computerised tomography (CT) renal tract imaging are used to both diagnose and stage the disease.

■ CT of chest and abdomen is used to detect metastases, and bone scintigraphy is performed in patients with bone pain or elevated alkaline phosphatase levels.

Symptoms and diagnosis of bladder cancer

More than 90% of bladder tumours are transitional cell carcinomas, ranging from well-differentiated lesions with little malignant potential to aggressive metastatic cancers. Although there has long been a view that there are superficial and invasive bladder cancers, it is now clear that the picture is more complex, with tumours of intermediate risk and variable behaviour. There were 8832 new registrations of bladder cancer in England in 2001 and 4412 deaths from bladder cancer in England and Wales in 2000.

Classification of bladder cancer

The tumour types seen in bladder cancer are shown in Table 1. In western countries, transitional cell carcinoma is by far the commonest type (95% of cases); in bilharzial areas such as Egypt, squamous cell cancer occurs commonly. Most bladder cancer is now attributable to cigarette smoking; although occupational causes due to exposure to chemicals have been identified, most of these agents are no longer used. The known environmental causes of bladder cancer are shown in Table 2.

Symptoms

The cardinal symptom of bladder cancer is *frank (macroscopic) haematuria*, although asymptomatic dipstick haematuria is also a common presentation. Bleeding is, typically, painless and occurs throughout the stream of urine; there may be clots and debris, the latter representing necrotic tumour or degenerate clot. Suprapubic, urethral or penile tip pain and lower urinary tract symptoms (frequency, urgency and nocturia) may be seen with solid tumours or with carcinoma in situ (malignant cystitis). Loin pain can occur when hydronephrosis results from an invasive tumour. Bladder tumours can cause hydronephrosis only by invasive obstruction of the ureter within the bladder; ureteric tumours or bladder tumours growing into the ureteric orifice, however, can obstruct the ureter to cause hydronephrosis by a bulk effect alone, even when superficial.

Examination

Examination rarely reveals any abnormality, although a palpable bladder may rarely be present if there are clots in the bladder, particularly if the patient presents urgently with bleeding and pain. The prostate should be assessed by rectal examination.

Investigation

Patients with haematuria are commonly investigated in the setting of a haematuria clinic. Urine should be cultured for infection, tested for proteinuria and a freshly voided specimen sent for cytological analysis. Malignant transitional cells in the urine (Fig. 1) are usually indicative of either high-grade papillary/solid tumours or of carcinoma in situ: positive urine cytology is uncommon in well-differentiated or moderately differentiated disease, which accounts for most cases of bladder cancer.

Imaging

Imaging of the upper tracts is performed to exclude hydronephrosis due to ureteric obstruction. Computerised tomography (CT) or magnetic resonance imaging (MRI) help to stage the local extent of bladder cancer and to detect regional lymphadenopathy when nodes are larger than 1 cm in diameter.

Cystoscopy

Most diagnostic cystoscopies are now performed on an outpatient or daycase basis, using a flexible cystoscope. This

Table 1 **Classification of bladder cancer**
Transitional cell carcinoma (95%)
Adenocarcinoma
Squamous cell carcinoma
Small cell carcinoma

Table 2 **Environmental causes of bladder cancer**	
Accepted	2-Naphthylamine
	4-Aminobiphenyl
	Benzidine
	N,N-bis-(2-chloroethyl)-2-naphthylamine
	4-Chlorotoluidine
	Schistosoma haematobium
	Phenacetin
	Cyclophosphamide
Suspected	Unsaturated aldehydes
	Nitrosamines
	4,4′-Methylene bis-(2-chloroaniline)
	o-Toluidine
Questionable	Caffeine
	Saccharine
	Cyclamate
	Tryptophan

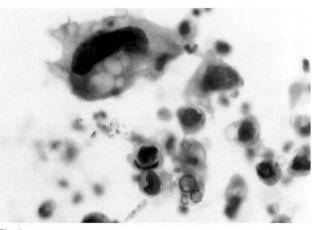

Fig. 1 **Abnormal urothelial cells in freshly voided urine.**

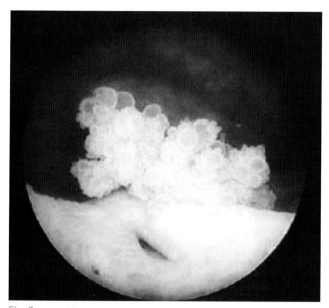

Fig. 2 **A papillary tumour of the bladder seen at cystoscopy.**

Table 3	**TNM staging of bladder cancer**	
Primary tumour (T)		
TX	Primary tumour cannot be assessed	
T0	No evidence of primary tumour	
Ta	Papillary tumour confined to urothelium	
TIS	Carcinoma in situ	
T1	Tumour invades lamina propria	
T2	Tumour invades detrusor muscle	
	T2a superficial muscle	
	T2b deep muscle	
T3	Tumour invades perivesical fat	
	T3a microscopically	
	T3b macroscopically	
T4	Tumour extends into prostate, uterus, vagina, pelvic side-wall or abdominal wall	
	T4a prostate, uterus or vagina	
	T4b pelvic side-wall or abdominal wall	
Regional lymph nodes (N)		
NX	Regional lymph nodes cannot be assessed	
N0	No tumour in lymph nodes	
N1	Single lymph node < 2 cm	
N2	One or more node 2–5 cm	
N3	One or more node > 5 cm	
Metastases (M)		
MX	Distant metastases cannot be assessed	
M0	No distant metastases	
M1	Distant metastases	

allows rapid examination of the urethra, prostatic fossa and bladder under local anaesthesia, minimising the impact of cystoscopy for the patient and allowing considerable numbers of patients to be assessed rapidly. If the bladder is normal, the patient can be reassured immediately. If a tumour is seen in the bladder (Fig. 2), it is easy to discuss the diagnosis and make plans for how to deal with it, tailored to the patient's particular circumstances, so that the patient knows what to expect next; resection of the tumour can then be scheduled appropriately.

Transurethral resection (TUR)/biopsy

Following the diagnosis of a new bladder tumour at flexible cystoscopy, resection of the tumour is arranged, either on a daycase basis (for small tumours) or as an inpatient. A resectoscope is used to resect the tumour from the bladder and to biopsy the underlying detrusor muscle layer. Skill is required to remove the tumour adequately without leaving a large defect in the bladder wall; in the intraperitoneal part (the vault) of the bladder, a full-thickness resection would result in intraperitoneal perforation and the need for open repair at

laparotomy. The resected tissue is submitted for histological assessment, where the pathologist confirms the diagnosis and allocates a stage and grade to the tumour.

Staging and grading of bladder cancer

The tumour/node/metastasis (TNM) classification of bladder tumours is shown in Table 3. After resection of the tumour, the prefix 'p' can be applied to the tumour stage (i.e. the pT stage). Nodal and metastatic staging is usually performed only in those patients with pT1 stage or greater. Nodes are staged using CT or MRI or, more definitively, following pelvic lymphadenectomy; metastases are staged using chest radiography, CT, MRI or bone scintigraphy.

Histopathological grading of the tumour is divided into three groups: G1, well differentiated; G2, moderately differentiated; G3, poorly differentiated. Both stage and grade govern the treatment options and ultimate prognosis.

> *Key points*
>
> ■ Most bladder cancer is now caused by cigarette smoking.
>
> ■ Haematuria is the cardinal symptom of bladder cancer.
>
> ■ Most bladder cancer is now diagnosed using a flexible cystoscopy under local anaesthetic.
>
> ■ Clinical staging and grading is performed following transurethral resection of the tumour and careful histopathological analysis.

Symptoms and diagnosis of prostate cancer

Prostate cancer is now the commonest solid tumour in men. In England and Wales each year, ~ 30 000 new patients are diagnosed and ~ 12 000 men die. It is apparently found less frequently in developing countries, mainly because there is no screening for early cancers by means of prostate-specific antigen (PSA) testing.

Epidemiology

There is a long preclinical phase, and the mean age at diagnosis for clinically presenting cancers is 72 years; it is rare in men under 50 years. The results of autopsy studies show small preclinical prostate cancers in 25% of men in their thirties and forties, 50% in their fifties and approximately 80% over 85 years. Clinically presenting prostate cancer is rare in the Far East but common in America and northern Europe, yet the incidence of latent cancer in these populations is the same. Environmental and dietary factors are important because migration of men from the Far East to America leads to an increased risk of prostate cancer in the migrating population, which, in the case of Japanese men, almost reaches the levels found in the white US population after two or three generations. Only 5–10% of cases of prostate cancer have a genetic influence, although the risk of prostate cancer increases with a family history of prostate cancer; the risk is sevenfold greater in patients with three first-degree relatives affected, especially if the cancer is diagnosed at a young age. The male relatives of *BRCA2* gene carriers are at increased risk of prostate cancer.

In England and Wales, prostate cancer is now the second commonest cause of male cancer death with approximately 12 500 deaths per year in the UK. The increased incidence of prostate cancer found during the 1990s in the USA coincided with the widespread adoption of PSA testing. Mortality from prostate cancer in the UK has not changed significantly in the last 10 years.

The lifetime risk of prostate cancer for a man in his fifties is in the region of 42%, but risk of death from prostate cancer is only 3%. There is a real risk of 'overdiagnosis' with PSA screening, with many low-risk prostate cancers being found that would not cause trouble to those men during their lifetime. It has been estimated that only one in five men diagnosed in screening studies would gain benefit from radical treatment. At present, it is not possible to identify which patients will have progressive disease and reduced life expectancy and, therefore, which require aggressive treatment. In England, because there is no screening programme ~ 40% of patients at diagnosis will have either locally advanced or metastatic disease.

Symptoms

There are no symptoms from the primary tumour in patients with early localised disease. Locally advanced cancers cause lower urinary tract symptoms (LUTS), but these are very common in men in their sixties and are most often due to benign prostatic hypertrophy (BPH). Eighty per cent of cancers arise from the peripheral zone (the outer part of the prostate), where they are unlikely to cause urinary symptoms. However, rapid progression of LUTS should raise suspicion of prostate cancer. The commonest site of metastases in prostate cancer is bone, and bone pain, pathological fracture or anaemia may be a presenting feature. The general effects of malignancy (cachexia, general malaise and weight loss) are seen only in patients with advanced disease.

Examination

Digital rectal examination (DRE) is essential to determine the clinical stage of the tumour. Because of PSA testing, most prostate cancers in the USA and Europe are clinically confined to the prostate at diagnosis. The tumour/node/metastasis (TNM) classification of prostate cancer is shown in Table 1.

Investigations

Prostate-specific antigen is a serine protease whose function is to liquefy semen. It is produced solely by the acini within the prostate, and its concentration is related to age, prostate volume and the presence of prostate cancer. PSA is not diagnostic of prostate cancer but, if the level is elevated above the age-adjusted range (Table 2) or associated with an abnormal DRE, further investigation by *transrectal ultrasound* and guided biopsies is needed. Transrectal ultrasound (TRUS) may provide staging information, but more reliable staging information is obtained from magnetic resonance imaging (MRI) or computerised tomography (CT) together with bone scintigraphy (Fig. 1).

In men in their sixties, 10% have a PSA of more than 3–4 ng/mL. Of these, 25% have prostate cancer, but ~ 15% of men with PSA levels between 2 and 3 (usually stated to be 'normal') have prostate cancer. PSA is neither sensitive nor specific in the diagnosis of early prostate cancer.

Pathology

Prostate cancers are adenocarcinomas and are graded using the *Gleason*

Table 1	**TNM staging of prostate cancer**
Primary tumour (T)	
TX	Primary tumour cannot be assessed
T0	No evidence of primary tumour
T1	Impalpable or not visible on imaging
	T1a incidental; present in < 5% of tissue
	T1b incidental; present in ≥ 5% of tissue
	T1c identified on needle biopsy
T2	Confined within the prostate
	T2a involving half a lobe or less
	T2b involving half a lobe
	T2c involving both lobes
T3	Extends through prostatic capsule
	T3a extends through one lobe
	T3b extends through both lobes
	T3c extends into seminal vesicles
T4	Involves structures other than seminal vesicle
	T4a involves bladder neck, external sphincter or rectum
	T4b involves muscles and/or rectal wall
Regional lymph nodes (N)	
NX	Regional lymph nodes cannot be assessed
N0	No tumour in lymph nodes
N1	Single lymph node < 2 cm
N2	One or more node 2–5 cm
N3	One or more node > 5 cm
Metastases (M)	
MX	Distant metastases cannot be assessed
M0	No distant metastases
M1	Distant metastases
	M1a bones(s) involved
	M1b other sites involved

Table 2	**Age-specific ranges for PSA**
Age (years)	**Maximum PSA(ng/mL)**
40–49	2.7
50–59	3.9
60–69	5.0
70–75	7.2

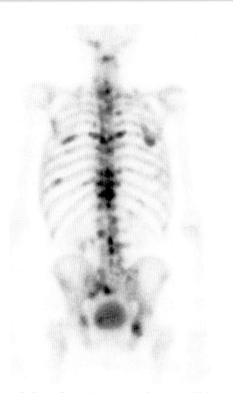

Fig. 1 **Bone scintigram in prostate cancer** showing multiple metastases in the axial skeleton.

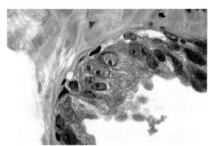

Fig. 3 **High-grade prostatic intraepithelial neoplasia** (PIN).

precursor of prostate cancer, and about 25% of men with PIN have associated prostate cancer on a later biopsy.

In patients who undergo prostatic biopsy for a raised PSA, 25% have an underlying cancer. Around 10 biopsies are taken under local anaesthesia by means of transrectal ultrasound guidance (TRUSP). The Gleason grading system assigns a score from 1 to 5 to the most common histological pattern and a second score to the next commonest pattern; the two scores are added together to produce the *Gleason sum score*; the Gleason sum score, therefore, ranges between 2 and 10 and is a useful prognostic indicator.

A number of nomograms may be used to predict the likelihood of extraprostatic extension, involvement of the seminal vesicles and the presence of nodal disease based on stage, grade and Gleason sum score. Patients with more poorly differentiated tumours (Gleason 8–10) are more likely to have nodal and metastatic disease at diagnosis and have greater risk of death from their tumour, whether actively treated or monitored.

grading system based on gland architecture and cellular morphology (Fig. 2). High-grade prostatic intraepithelial neoplasia (PIN) has the cellular appearance of cancer, but the basement membrane is intact (Fig. 3); this is thought to be a

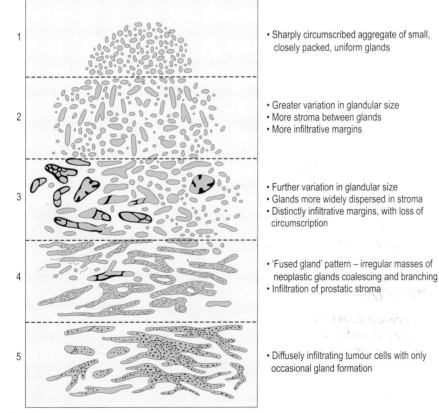

- Sharply circumscribed aggregate of small, closely packed, uniform glands

- Greater variation in glandular size
- More stroma between glands
- More infiltrative margins

- Further variation in glandular size
- Glands more widely dispersed in stroma
- Distinctly infiltrative margins, with loss of circumscription

- 'Fused gland' pattern – irregular masses of neoplastic glands coalescing and branching
- Infiltration of prostatic stroma

- Diffusely infiltrating tumour cells with only occasional gland formation

Fig. 2 **Gleason grading system** for prostate cancer.

> ## *Key points*
>
> - The incidence of prostate cancer is increasing, but there is no clear evidence that radical treatment will lead to an overall reduction in mortality.
>
> - In screen-detected cancers, only 20% of cases will gain benefit from radical treatment.
>
> - An abnormal digital rectal examination and/or prostate-specific antigen (PSA) elevation are the main indicators for carrying out prostatic ultrasound and prostatic biopsy (TRUSP).
>
> - The complication rate of TRUSP is low, but a negative result does not exclude a cancer, and 20–35% of patients will have cancer identified on subsequent biopsy.
>
> - High-grade prostatic intraepithelial neoplasia (PIN) is an indication for repeat prostatic biopsy as there is a greater risk of multifocal prostate cancer in the region of 25–35% of cases undergoing repeat prostatic biopsy.
>
> - ~ 50% of prostate cancers are localised to the prostate at diagnosis.

Prostate cancer treatment

Fifty per cent of patients have organ-confined disease at presentation and are suitable for radical treatment; in locally advanced disease or metastatic disease, palliative care is all that can be offered.

Treatment of localised disease

The main options available for localised disease are active monitoring, radiotherapy and radical prostatectomy; there have been no randomised controlled trials comparing these. As a result, when a patient is diagnosed with localised prostate cancer, there is no clear direction as to the most effective treatment. Many clinicians therefore allow the patient to participate in management decisions based chiefly on a discussion of potential side-effects.

Active monitoring
This involves no active treatment but repeated measurement of prostate-specific antigen (PSA) levels with intervention only if the PSA rises significantly. The natural history of prostate cancer is long, and many patients diagnosed with prostate cancer will die with their cancer and not from it, especially if they are elderly and have accompanying comorbidities such as ischaemic heart disease, hypertension or diabetes. In younger patients with high-grade disease, active monitoring is not appropriate because the likelihood of progression is high and, once the disease has metastasised, cure is no longer achievable.

Radical radiotherapy
Radiotherapy can be delivered to the prostate from outside the body (external beam radiotherapy) or by the introduction of radioactive seeds directly into the prostate. External beam radiotherapy is generally preceded by 3 months of chemical castration using a luteinising hormone-releasing hormone

(LHRH) agonist; this is continued during the treatment, which is spread over a 7-week period and delivers a total radiation dose of 70 Gy.

Conformal radiotherapy, in which treatment is confined to the prostate and seminal vesicles, sparing neighbouring structures (bladder and rectum), enables higher doses to be given, and the increased precision results in fewer local side-effects (cystitis and radiation proctitis). Incontinence is rare, although a small proportion may develop urethral strictures; erectile dysfunction (impotence) is seen in 40–50% of patients due to radiation injury to the neurovascular bundles. Five per cent of patients have radiation proctitis 1 year after completing radiotherapy. Lack of accurate staging despite cross-sectional imaging and the inability to deliver a lethal radiation dose to the tumour may lead to radiation failure, but patients with comorbidities can undergo this treatment provided they have a projected life expectancy of 10 years or more.

Brachytherapy involves placement of radioactive seeds within the prostate under ultrasound control (Fig. 1). The radioactive source is either ^{125}iodine or ^{103}palladium, and seeds are inserted under ultrasound guidance. Patients with large prostates (> 50 mL) are generally not considered for this technique due to inability to place the seeds to irradiate the entire gland. In addition, the side-effects of storage bladder symptoms and urinary retention are more likely in patients with larger prostates. Accurate placement of the radioactive seeds causes less rectal and neurovascular bundle toxicity. Patients with smaller, less aggressive tumours respond better, and this makes it difficult to compare external beam radiotherapy with brachytherapy.

Radical prostatectomy
If prostate cancer is localised to the gland, cure can be achieved by radical prostatectomy, in which the entire prostate and both

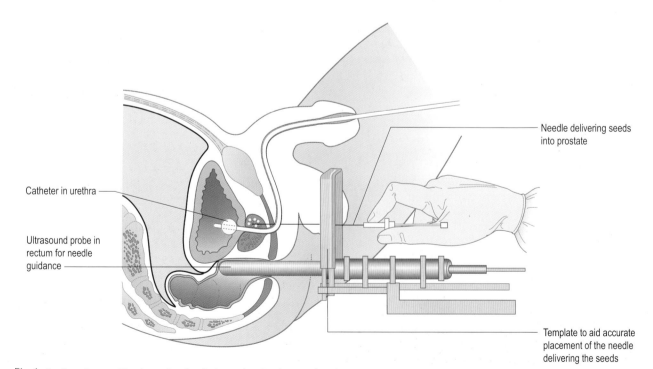

Catheter in urethra

Ultrasound probe in rectum for needle guidance

Needle delivering seeds into prostate

Template to aid accurate placement of the needle delivering the seeds

Fig. 1 **Radioactive seed implantation** (brachytherapy) under ultrasound guidance.

seminal vesicles are excised with pelvic lymph node sampling. The main advantage of this technique is that a clearer prognosis is known because accurate staging and grading are available from the histopathology (Fig. 2). Post-operatively, any detectable PSA is a clear indication of treatment failure from either persistent or recurrent disease.

Surgical techniques have improved considerably over the last 15 years with a move towards minimally invasive surgery, using laparoscopy and, more recently, robot-assisted laparoscopy. The latter technique enables greater control of laparoscopic instruments by a surgeon who operates remotely from the patient at a control console (Fig. 3). The main side-effects of radical prostatectomy are impotence (in 10–90%); higher rates are seen when preoperative potency is reduced and when the neurovascular bundles cannot be preserved during surgery. With minimally invasive techniques, there is a greater likelihood that neurovascular bundle preservation can be achieved.

The other main side-effect is incontinence of urine, which affects 2–30% of patients. Care must be taken to preserve the distal sphincter during surgery, and preparing patients preoperatively with pelvic floor exercises is important. Long-term incontinence, requiring pads or other appliances, occurs in 2–5% of cases. Stenosis at the vesicourethral anastomosis develops in 5–10%.

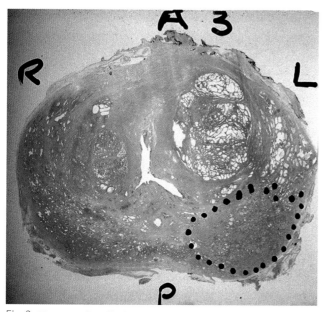

Fig. 2 **Macroscopic radical prostatectomy specimen** prepared for histological assessment.

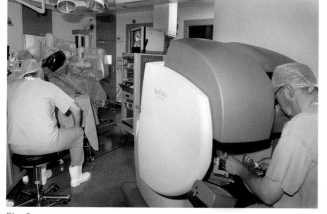

Fig. 3 **Radical robotic-assisted laparoscopic prostatectomy.**

Locally advanced or metastatic disease

Ninety per cent of tumours are hormone dependent or sensitive, at least initially. Hormone therapy remains the mainstay of treatment for advanced disease but, in elderly patients with localised disease, it may also be a reasonable alternative. While hormone therapy may not offer improved life expectancy, it may reduce complications from disease progression.

In locally advanced disease, where the tumour extends beyond the prostate capsule or into the seminal vesicles but has not metastasised, a combination of hormone therapy and radiotherapy is the mainstay of treatment. There is little place for surgery in locally advanced disease, except in young patients, but radiotherapy can be used after surgery if it has proved impossible to eradicate the tumour completely.

Patients with metastatic disease have a shortened life expectancy. The mainstay of treatment is hormone therapy by androgen deprivation using either *LHRH agonist injections*, *antiandrogen tablets* or bilateral *orchidectomy*. The first option is most commonly used but, because the first LHRH agonist injection causes a rise in testosterone and may cause 'tumour flare', oral antiandrogens are used for 2 weeks prior to injection. The main side-effects are hot flushes, loss of libido, impotence, weight gain, gynaecomastia and osteoporosis. There is a survival advantage if metastatic disease is treated with hormone therapy, but hormone therapy can never cure the patients and is intended primarily to reduce complications. The average response to hormone therapy lasts 2 years, after which the introduction of antiandrogens or stilbestrol or bilateral orchidectomy may produce a further response.

Treatment response is monitored by PSA levels and, despite its diagnostic limitations, PSA is a sensitive marker of tumour progression or recurrence during follow-up. The effectiveness of any treatment is easily gauged by the nadir level of PSA and failure in the rate of rise in PSA.

Minimally invasive treatments

Minimally invasive treatments are being used for primary disease or after failure of first-line therapy, but there is no clear evidence of their efficacy from randomised controlled trials. *High-intensity focused ultrasound* is delivered through the rectum and has the potential to cause rectal fistulae. *Cryotherapy* is delivered transperineally, in a similar way to brachytherapy, and may have a place in radiation failure; impotence occurs in 100%, and the risk of fistula formation is also high.

Key points

- It is unclear which localised prostate cancers require treatment, and the choice is often made by the patient based on treatment side-effects.

- There are no randomised controlled trials available to provide evidence for the most appropriate treatment in localised disease, but studies are currently taking place.

- There is an increasing drive towards minimally invasive treatment with fewer side-effects, and this may lead to the overtreatment of patients.

- In locally advanced disease, radiotherapy and hormone therapy are the mainstay of treatment, although young patients may benefit from surgery and adjuvant radiotherapy or hormone therapy.

- Hormone therapy is the mainstay of treatment of metastatic disease but provides only palliation.

Penile cancer

Penile cancer is uncommon in developed countries and occurs only in uncircumcised men.

Incidence

The highest incidence is seen in Africa, Asia and South America, but penile cancer is rare in Europe, affecting only 1 in 100 000 men. Ninety-five per cent of penile cancers are squamous cell carcinomas (Fig. 1), with the remainder being melanomas, basal cell carcinomas or lymphomas. Neonatal circumcision has a protective effect. Cancer affects the prepuce alone in 25% and the glans penis alone in 50%; it is unusual for the penile shaft to be involved.

Premalignant abnormalities

Human papillomavirus (HPV) 16 and 18 are most commonly associated with genital cancers. HPV-16 DNA has been found in 50% of penile cancers or areas of dysplasia. *Erythroplasia of Queyrat, Bowen's disease* and *bowenoid papulosis* are believed to be premalignant lesions.

Clinical findings

The vast majority of patients with penile cancer are uncircumcised and have a mass visible or palpable beneath the prepuce (Fig. 2). Inguinal lymphadenopathy is present in 60% of patients at presentation, often due to secondary infection. However, 20% of patients with impalpable lymph nodes have nodal micrometastases.

Diagnosis

Circumcision with biopsy is the mainstay of diagnosis and is essential before treatment. The primary lesion is staged by clinical examination, although ultrasound or magnetic resonance imaging (MRI) may be useful to assess the involvement of the corpora cavernosum. The tumour/node/metastasis (TNM) classification of penile cancer is shown in Table 1. Following initial biopsy, *dynamic scintigraphy* and *sentinel lymph node biopsy* may be performed in high-risk disease (Table 2) to prevent unnecessary lymphadenectomy.

Assessment of lymph nodes at diagnosis

Fifty-five per cent of palpable lymph nodes are reactive at diagnosis. Close surveillance of palpable lymph nodes after antibiotic therapy is the favoured approach for low-risk disease (Table 2). If nodes persist after this, biopsies (aspiration, core or open) may be necessary. If the inguinal nodes do contain tumour, abdominal and chest computerised tomography (CT) are performed. Bone scintigraphy is indicated only when symptomatic bone pain is present.

Management of the primary tumour

The management of the primary tumour remains controversial. While the aim is to remove the primary tumour, there is increasing interest in conservative surgery to maintain cosmetic appearance with normal sexual and urinary function.

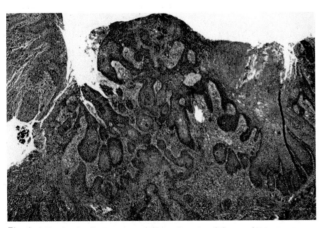

Fig. 1 **Histology of squamous cell carcinoma of the penis.**

Table 1 **TNM classification of penile cancer**

Primary tumour (T)	
Tx	Primary tumour cannot be assessed
T0	No evidence of primary tumour
TIS	Carcinoma in situ
Ta	Non-invasive verrucous carcinoma
T1	Tumour invades subepithelial connective tissue
T2	Tumour invades corpus spongiosum or cavernosum
T3	Tumour invades urethra or prostate
T4	Tumour invades other adjacent structures
Lymph nodes (N)	
Nx	Regional lymph nodes cannot be assessed
N0	No evidence of lymph node metastases
N1	Metastasis in single inguinal lymph node
N2	Metastasis in multiple or bilateral superficial lymph nodes
N3	Metastasis in deep inguinal or pelvic lymph nodes, unilateral or bilateral
Metastases (M)	
Mx	Distant metastases cannot be assessed
M0	No evidence of distant metastases
M1	Distant metastases

Table 2 **Risk stratification after staging of penile cancer**

Clinical stage	Recurrence risk
pTIS	Low
pTa grade 1 or 2	
pT1 grade 1	
pT1 grade 2	Intermediate
Greater than pT2	High
Any stage grade 3	

Low and intermediate risk

Treatment options include laser therapy, cryotherapy, photodynamic therapy, topical chemotherapy (5-fluorouracil cream), radiotherapy, brachytherapy and surgery (partial penectomy or glansectomy). When follow-up is likely to be suboptimal, radical surgery is usually advised. External beam radiotherapy and brachytherapy produce complete response rates of 56% and 70% respectively; common complications include telangiectasia (90%), urethral stricture (35%) and meatal stenosis (15–30%). The local recurrence rate is similar for all treatment modalities (15–25%).

High risk

Radical surgery is required (partial or total amputation dependent on the local extent of disease).

Local disease recurrence

Partial or total amputation is recommended unless there is no proven invasion into the corpus cavernosum, when further use of a conservative option may be justified.

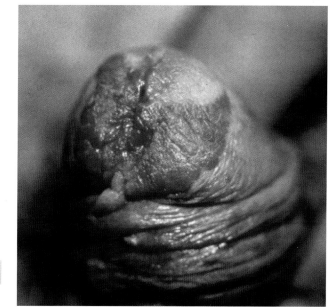

Fig. 2 **Carcinoma of glans penis** at presentation.

Management of lymph nodes

Impalpable lymph nodes

In low-risk patients, nodal micrometastases occur in < 20%, and surveillance is the optimum measure; if surveillance is likely to be inadequate, a modified inguinal lymphadenectomy is performed. This has a lower morbidity than more radical lymphadenectomy.

In intermediate-risk patients, dynamic sentinel node scintigraphy and node sampling are useful with modified lymphadenectomy if the nodes are positive.

In high-risk patients, occult nodal metastases are seen in 70%. Modified lymphadenectomy should be performed but, if frozen section sampling during the procedure reveals positive nodes, the procedure should be converted to a radical lymphadenectomy.

Palpable lymph nodes

Palpable lymph nodes after antibiotic therapy, confirmed to contain tumour by fine needle or core biopsy, should be managed by radical inguinal lymphadenectomy. Although post-operative morbidity is high, cure is possible in 15–55% of patients.

Fixed inguinal lymph nodes

These are managed by neoadjuvant chemotherapy followed by radical inguinal lymphadenectomy.

Palpable inguinal nodes after primary treatment

Bilateral radical inguinal lymphadenectomy is usually recommended as contralateral nodal involvement is seen in 30%. However, if patients develop unilateral lymphadenopathy after a long interval and no more than a single node contains metastatic tumour, the risk of contralateral recurrence is only 10% and further surveillance may be advised. The main risks of radical inguinal lymphadenectomy are skin flap necrosis, lymphoedema, seroma formation, deep venous thrombosis and pulmonary embolism.

Advanced disease

Neoadjuvant chemotherapy may be indicated before surgery for fixed inguinal lymph nodes, using a platinum-based drug and 5-fluorouracil; response rates of 70% are seen with survival rates of 23%. Similar regimes are also used in advanced disease with a complete or partial response in 30%.

Key points

- Penile cancer is uncommon in developed countries and occurs only in uncircumcised men.
- The human papillomavirus (HPV-16 and -18) is associated with 50% of cases of penile cancer.
- There has been a trend towards organ-preserving surgery to preserve function and cosmesis, but the achievement of negative surgical margins is essential.
- Based on TNM classification, patients can be grouped into low, intermediate and high risk.
- 60% of patients have palpable lymph nodes at diagnosis, but only 45% have nodal tumour because coexisting infection is common.
- Modified or radical inguinal lymphadenectomy may be necessary to diagnose and excise metastatic nodal disease and may achieve a cure.

Tumours of the testis and scrotum

Testicular tumours

Incidence and aetiology

Testicular cancer is the commonest malignancy in 15- to 35-year-old men but makes up only 1–2% of all male cancers. Two per cent of affected patients have an affected family member, and 80% of invasive tumours have an extra copy of the 12p chromosome. Several factors are known to predispose to testicular cancer (Table 1). Most patients present in the third or fourth decades, but spermatocytic seminoma and lymphoma occur in older men.

Pathology

Some 90–95% of tumours arise from germ cells; germ cells are more prone to DNA mutations than supporting cells because they are mitotically active. The main histological types are seminomatous and non-seminomatous (Table 2). Testicular cancer spreads by direct infiltration into adjacent scrotal structures, via the lymphatics to para-aortic nodes and via the bloodstream.

Clinical features and investigation

The usual presentation is with painless, unilateral scrotal enlargement (Fig. 1). Twenty per cent of patients give a history of scrotal trauma, which may obscure the initial diagnosis. Presentation is often delayed by the patient, and this adversely affects prognosis. Symptoms from metastases are rare, but gynaecomastia is seen in 2%. Examination of the scrotum reveals a mass in the body of the testis, although a secondary hydrocele may render the testis impalpable. The diagnosis is confirmed by scrotal ultrasound, which shows a mass in the body of the testis. Tumour markers (Table 3) may help in diagnosis but are more useful for monitoring response to treatment and for determining whether patients fall into a good, intermediate or poor prognostic group.

Surgical management

Treatment is by radical orchidectomy via an inguinal approach to avoid contaminating the scrotal lymphatic drainage; even if

Table 1 **Factors predisposing to testicular cancer**	
Cryptorchidism	Accounts for 10% of all cancers and increases the risk of malignancy 30- to 50-fold. Some 5–10% develop cancer in the contralateral (normally descended) testis
Intratubular germ cell neoplasia	50% develop invasive cancer within 5 years
Familial	First-degree relatives have a 6- to 10-fold increased risk
Infertility	Abnormal testes (especially with raised follicle-stimulating hormone) have increased risk
Previous testicular tumour	5% develop a second primary tumour
Testicular microcalcification	Seen in association with testicular cancer and in damaged testes; malignant potential unknown

Table 2 **Histological types of testicular tumour**
Germ cell tumours
Seminomatous (35–40%)
Classic seminoma
Spermatocytic seminoma
Non-seminomatous (50–55%)
Embryonal carcinoma
Yolk sac (endodermal sinus) tumour
Trophoblastic tumour (choriocarcinoma)
Teratoma
Non-germ cell tumours
Sex cord and stromal tumours
Leydig (interstitial) cell tumours (1–3%)
Sertoli–mesenchymal tumours (< 1%)
Large cell tumour
Granulosa cell tumours
Theca cell tumours
Sex cord stromal tumours
Gonadoblastoma
Miscellaneous tumours
Hamartomas
Carcinoid tumours
Benign tumours (epidermoid)
Lymphoid and haemopoietic tumours (5%)
Metastases
Prostate, lung, colon, kidney

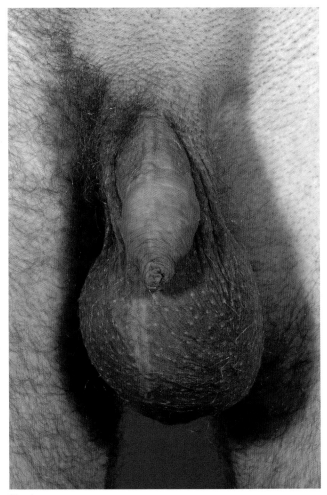

Fig. 1 **Unilateral scrotal swelling due to testicular cancer.**

Table 3 **Tumour markers for testicular cancer**	
Tumour marker	**Sensitivity**
α-Fetoprotein (AFP)	Raised in 90% of seminoma
β-Human chorionic gonadotrophins (HCG)	Raised in 80% of embryonal cancer and in trophoblastic tumours
Lactate dehydrogenase (LDH)	Raised in some seminomas and non-seminomatous tumours; limited use
Placental alkaline phosphatase (PLAP)	Raised in up to 35% of the normal population (especially smokers); limited use

metastases are present, the testis should be removed because the primary tumour does not respond effectively to chemotherapy. Sperm banking and preservation is offered to all patients, and a prosthetic testis may be inserted at the time of surgery. There remains some debate about the need to biopsy the contralateral testis to exclude *carcinoma in situ* (Fig. 2).

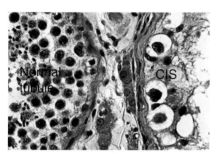

Fig. 2 **Intratubular germ cell neoplasia** (carcinoma in situ, CIS).

Oncological management

Once the histological type has been confirmed, oncological referral is needed for clinical staging (Fig. 3) using computerised tomography (CT) of the abdomen and chest.

Standard therapy for stage I seminomatous germ cell tumours is low-dose radiotherapy to the para-aortic nodes, which results in cure rates of almost 100%; higher stages are treated with chemotherapy.

For stage I non-seminomatous germ cell tumours, chemotherapy is used because of a 28% relapse rate without adjuvant treatment; higher stages are treated with chemotherapy. Chemotherapy regimens vary but usually involve multiple drugs (e.g. bleomycin, etoposide, carboplatin) given in cycles at 3-weekly intervals. Lymphoid and haemopoietic tumours are treated with appropriate chemotherapy. Morbidity from chemotherapy is significant (e.g. neutropenic sepsis), and complications may be life-threatening. Carcinoma in situ of the contralateral testis may be treated by local radiotherapy or orchidectomy.

Prognosis

Stage I disease can usually be cured in all patients. In higher stage disease, complete remission is seen in 80–90% of patients. In patients who do not respond and in the 10% who relapse after chemotherapy, second-line chemotherapy may be used (with autologous bone marrow transplantation or peripheral blood stem cell support as needed), but such patients usually undergo radical retroperitoneal node excision; 60% are found to have residual node malignancy.

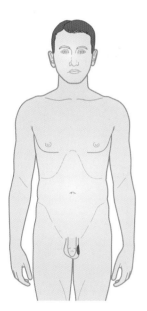

Stage I – Disease confined to testes

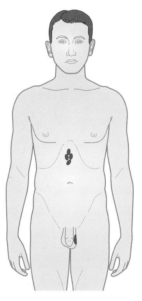

Stage II – Infradiaphragmatic node involvement
A: <2 cm
B: 2–5 cm
C: >5 cm

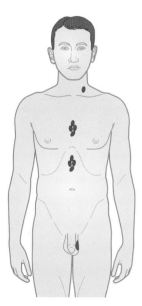

Stage III – Supradiaphragmatic node involvement

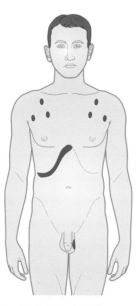

Stage IV – Extralymphatic disease

Fig. 3 **Clinical staging of testicular cancer.**

Scrotal tumours

Squamous carcinoma of the scrotal skin is now very rare except in those exposed to exogenous carcinogens (e.g. soot, machine oil). Early invasion of the scrotal contents and inguinal nodes is common. Treatment is by wide local excision, skin grafting and block dissection of affected lymph nodes.

Key points

- Testicular cancer is the commonest male cancer in the third and fourth decades.
- There are several well-known predispositions, especially cryptorchidism, carcinoma in situ and a previous testicular tumour.
- Surgical excision followed by radiotherapy or chemotherapy cures almost all patients even when the cancer has spread.
- Relapse or recurrence is uncommon and is managed by second-line chemotherapy or surgical node excision.

Benign Genital Disorders

Benign disorders of the penis

While the skin of the penis may be affected by a variety of generalised dermatological conditions (see pp. 138 and 139), there are a number of benign disorders specific to the penis.

Phimosis

The foreskin normally begins to separate from the glans penis, progressing from proximal to distal, from the age of 5 years. Ninety-five per cent of non-retractile foreskins become retractile around the time of puberty and do not require surgical intervention. Failure of separation may result in preputial adhesions, although most adhesions separate spontaneously with increasing age. Phimosis is a pathological condition in which the foreskin is so tight that it cannot be fully retracted over the glans. It should be distinguished from the non-retractile foreskin normally seen in infancy. Most cases of phimosis are idiopathic in origin, but tightness of the foreskin may be caused by balanitis xerotica obliterans (BXO, Fig. 1), chronic balanitis and post-traumatic cicatrisation.

Clinical presentation

Children with phimosis usually present with ballooning of the foreskin (Fig. 2). Ballooning promotes washout of smegma and is not a problem unless associated with recurrent balanitis. Adults may notice that the foreskin no longer fully retracts or that their urinary stream is constricted. Phimosis may also be associated with an underlying penile cancer, and this is sometimes visible or palpable behind the foreskin.

Management

Treatment in children is initially directed at eliminating infection by the use of systemic or topical antibiotics; circumcision or prepuceplasty may be necessary once the infection has settled. In adults, circumcision is usually required, but prepuceplasty is ineffective.

Paraphimosis

Paraphimosis occurs when the foreskin is retracted over the glans but cannot be returned to its normal position. It occurs with an erect penis, but is also seen after catheterisation or urethral instrumentation when the foreskin is retracted for cleaning but is not replaced at the end of the procedure. The foreskin becomes painful, swollen and impossible to replace over the glans (Fig. 3).

Management

In the early stages, it is possible to reduce the paraphimosis by squeezing and elongating the oedematous tissues, under local

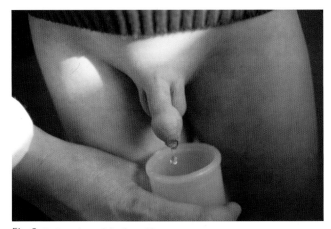

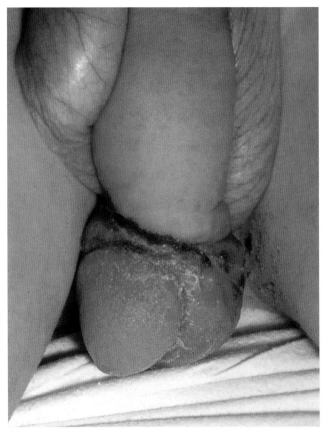

Fig. 2 **Ballooning of the foreskin.**

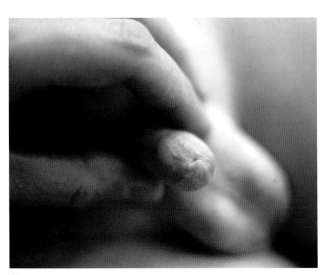

Fig. 1 **Phimosis due to balanitis xerotica obliterans** (BXO).

Fig. 3 **Paraphimosis.**

Table 1	**Types of priapism**		
Type	**Clinical features**	**Causes**
Low-flow (veno-occlusive)	Painful, rigid, no response to sex Contains dark, acidotic blood pH < 7.25, po_2 < 4, pco_2 > 8	Drugs (injected prostaglandins, psychotropic drugs, marijuana) Blood disorders (leukaemia, myeloma, sickle cell disease) Miscellaneous (carbon monoxide poisoning, rabies, spinal stenosis) Metabolic problems (amyloid, gout) Idiopathic (in 33%)
'Stuttering' (veno-occlusive)	As above	Drugs (psychotropic drugs, anticoagulants)
High-flow (arteriocavernous fistula)	Less painful, semirigid, responds to sex Contains red, oxygenated blood pH > 7.25, po_2 > 4, pco_2 < 8	Blunt, pelvic trauma Needlestick injury during penile injection

anaesthetic penile block, and then sliding the foreskin over the glans. If this fails, an emergency dorsal slit or circumcision may be necessary. After successful reduction of a paraphimosis, elective circumcision is often necessary to prevent recurrence.

Priapism

Priapism is a prolonged painful erection not associated with sexual desire. The types of priapism are shown in Table 1. Typically, the corpus spongiosum is flaccid, while the corpora cavernosa are erect (Fig. 4).

Clinical management
Low-flow priapism produces hypercapnia and irreversible, painful muscle necrosis within 24 h, resulting in impotence in 100%, so urgent treatment is needed. Wide-bore cannulae inserted into the corpora cavernosa are used to irrigate the penis with saline; if unsuccessful, an α-adrenergic agonist such as phenylephrine (250–500 µg) is injected to produce muscle constriction. If the priapism fails to deflate, shunting is no longer considered to be worthwhile, and penile prostheses should be inserted once the acute phase has resolved. Any underlying predisposition should also be treated aggressively and contributory drugs withdrawn.

Stuttering priapism is managed as above, and recurrences may be prevented using terbutaline, phenylpropanolamine, digoxin or a luteinising hormone-releasing hormone (LHRH) agonist.

High-flow priapism should be investigated by pelvic angiography with embolisation of any fistulae between the cavernous artery and the corpora cavernosa. The risk of impotence is lower (up to 20%) in high-flow priapism.

Peyronie's disease

This is a fibrotic process of unknown cause that affects Buck's fascia and the corpora cavernosa in up to 3% of men. Repeated coital trauma may be the precipitating cause. Initially, pain is often felt with an inflammatory mass in the penis. This inflammatory stage (which lasts up to 3 months) then settles, and healing with scarring results in fibrosis, causing angulation of the penis on erection (usually up towards the abdomen). An induration or plaque of fibrosis is palpable in the penis, and 30% of cases are associated with Dupuytren's contracture. In cases of diagnostic doubt, a cavernosogram with injected prostaglandin E2 (alprostadil) may be performed.

Management
Peyronie's disease resolves spontaneously in 60–70% of patients over 12–18 months so the majority of patients require no active treatment. Medical treatment is ineffective, but tamoxifen (25 mg daily for 6 weeks) may reduce pain in the

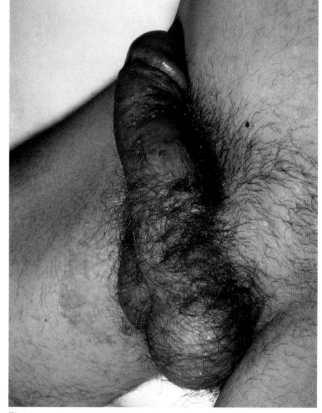

Fig. 4 **Priapism.**

inflammatory stage and minimise any subsequent angulation. Low-energy shock wave treatment to disperse the plaque sometimes gives good results.

Surgery to straighten the penis is only indicated when the erectile deformity prevents intercourse; penile prostheses may be required if the disease is so extensive that it prevents full tumescence. A surgical approach should be undertaken only when the deformity has been stable for at least 6 months, and patients should be warned about potential surgical complications of impotence, penile shortening, loss of penile sensation and palpable sutures within the penis.

> ### Key points
>
> - Phimosis is a pathological condition in which the foreskin cannot be fully retracted due to scarring of the foreskin.
>
> - Paraphimosis is due to retraction of a tight foreskin over an erect glans penis, after which the foreskin cannot be replaced.
>
> - Priapism is a urological emergency; delayed treatment (after 24 h) may result in impotence, especially with low-flow priapism.
>
> - Peyronie's disease is a self-limiting condition in most men; corrective surgery is indicated if the degree of angulation prevents intercourse and the disease has been stable for at least 6 months.

Diseases of the genital skin

General assessment

The spectrum of genital skin disease is shown in Table 1. A definitive diagnosis can usually be made on the history and examination alone. Examination of the regional lymph nodes and extragenital sites is essential, although lesional biopsy may be necessary to confirm the diagnosis.

Fournier's gangrene

This is a destructive infection originating from the skin, urethra or perianal area. Many organisms have been implicated (both facultative and anaerobic), and patients often have a history of diabetes, recent trauma, urethral instrumentation, anorectal sepsis or urethral stricture. The initial picture is of localised cellulitis, which progresses rapidly to destructive necrosis with systemic toxicity. Progression is rapid and, if untreated, the mortality rate is 100%.

Management is by intravenous fluid replacement and broad-spectrum antibiotics with immediate debridement of all necrotic tissue (Fig. 1). Urinary diversion by suprapubic catheterisation is often necessary and, at a later stage, skin grafts may be required if the debrided areas do not heal by first intention. Aggressive treatment reduces the mortality to 20%.

Contact dermatitis

Genital skin lesions may be induced by soaps, cosmetics, condoms, contraceptive jellies, topical agents and plants (e.g. poison ivy). Management involves avoidance of the suspected agent, application of moist dressings and topical steroids.

Fixed drug eruptions

These are well-defined lesions that recur at the same site with every exposure to the offending drug. They appear as raised, erythematous patches that may later vesiculate or ulcerate. Implicated drugs include tetracycline, sulphonamides, co-trimoxazole and barbiturates. Management involves local toilet and cessation of the responsible drug.

Factitious dermatitis

This may appear in a number of different ways, including infection. It is due to self-mutilation, scratching, blunt trauma, application of heat/cold or caustic substances. There is usually an underlying psychiatric problem that requires specialist assessment.

Psoriasis

Psoriasis is a common, chronic inflammatory condition that can occur at any age. It most commonly affects extensor surfaces as red plaques with silvery scales. The groin and perianal cleft are often affected, and solitary plaques may appear on the shaft of the penis. The diagnosis can usually be made by finding other areas of involvement (e.g. the scalp, elbows, knees, nails). Management is dermatological but, for penile lesions, topical hydrocortisone cream may be effective.

Table 1 **Genital skin diseases**	
Infective	Sexually transmitted disease (see pp. 38 and 39)
	Fournier's gangrene
	Parasitic: scabies, pubic lice (common); amoebiasis, Leishmaniasis (rare)
Exogenous	Contact dermatitis
	Fixed drug eruption
	Factitious
Inflammatory	Psoriasis
	Seborrhoeic dermatitis
	Lichen planus
	Zoon's balanitis
	Balanitis xerotica obliterans (BXO)
	Multisystem: Reiter's, Behçet's, Crohn's
Benign tumours	Pearly penile papules
	Sebaceous cyst
	Haemangioma
	Pigmented naevi
	Neurofibroma
Premalignant	Erythroplasia of Queyrat
	Bowen's disease
	Paget's disease
Malignant tumours	Squamous cell carcinoma
	Malignant melanoma
	Kaposi's sarcoma

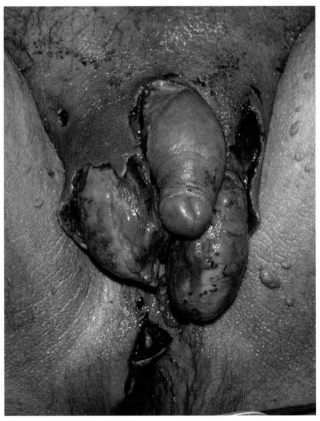

Fig. 1 **Fournier's scrotal gangrene** after surgical debridement.

Seborrhoeic dermatitis

This appears as scaly red patches with mild pruritis, and the differential diagnosis includes psoriasis. Extragenital disease usually involves the scalp, brows, cheeks and chest. Treatment is with topical steroids.

Lichen planus

This is an inflammatory condition of unknown aetiology that can occur at any age. Lesions tend to occur on the glans penis in men and on the labia or introitus in women. Typically, these are violaceous papules with white streaks (*Wickham's striae*). While oral lichen planus has been associated with malignancy, genital lichen planus has not. Pruritus is usually the main symptom, and treatment is with topical or systemic steroids.

Zoon's balanitis (plasma cell balanitis)

This tends to occur in middle-aged and elderly, uncircumcised men affecting the glans and prepuce. The lesions are usually painless, shiny, moist and well defined (Fig. 2). Biopsy is often required to exclude other diagnoses and shows a dense plasma cell infiltrate. Treatment involves keeping the affected areas dry and the use of topical steroids; circumcision may be required if topical treatment fails.

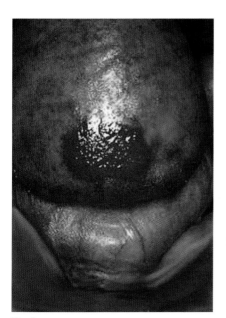

Fig. 2 **Plasma cell balanitis.**

Balanitis xerotica obliterans (BXO)

This is an inflammatory condition of unknown aetiology, occurring most commonly in middle-aged, uncircumcised men. The lesions appear as irregular, flat, pale patches on the foreskin or glans penis. The foreskin becomes indurated and thickened with preputial stenosis; it may also stenose the urethral meatus and spread into the fossa navicularis of the urethra. Topical steroids are often effective, but circumcision is usually indicated for a phimosis. If meatal stenosis develops, repeated dilatation or meatoplasty may be needed, and resistant, chronic disease may require excision with skin grafting.

Behçet's syndrome

This is a recurrent, systemic disease of unknown cause in which 60–90% of patients develop punched-out genital ulcers. These are usually multiple and painful, situated on the scrotum, penis or groin in men and the vulva, vagina and groin in women. Associated symptoms include oral ulcers, erythema nodosum, iritis/uveitis, oligoarthritis and gastrointestinal symptoms. Diagnosis is made from non-genital manifestations and by excluding other causes of genital ulcers (see pp. 38 and 39). Local treatment with topical steroids is effective but, for systemic disease, treatment with oral steroids, dapsone, methotrexate, non-steroidal anti-inflammatory drugs (NSAIDs), azathioprine or ciclosporin may be needed.

Benign tumours

Pearly penile papules are common. They are usually found at the coronal margin

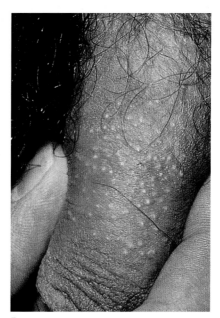

Fig. 3 **Multiple sebaceous cysts** (milia) in ectopic sebaceous glands on the penile shaft.

or on the frenulum. Their characteristic appearance and position are usually diagnostic, and no treatment is required.

Sebaceous cysts are found anywhere where there are sebaceous glands. They are commonly multiple and usually occur on the scrotal skin. Cysts of ectopic sebaceous glands may be found on the prepuce and the shaft of the penis (Fig. 3). No treatment is required, but scrotal cysts may be excised to improve cosmetic appearances.

Haemangiomas are usually found on the glans penis. They require no treatment and tend to regress spontaneously.

Pigmented naevi may occur on the genitalia. Biopsy is often needed to exclude malignant melanoma or Kaposi's sarcoma.

> ### Key points
>
> - Accurate diagnosis of genital skin lesions can usually be made from the history and examination alone.
> - Fournier's gangrene is a highly aggressive infection that requires urgent surgical debridement and broad-spectrum antibiotics.
> - Exogenous factors such as chemicals, drugs and deliberate self-harm should always be considered.
> - Inflammatory conditions may require biopsy to confirm the diagnosis, but local treatment is usually effective.
> - Benign tumours may be removed for cosmetic reasons.

Scrotal swellings

True scrotal swellings can be divided into four main groups; cystic, solid, inflammatory and miscellaneous (Table 1). Careful examination of the scrotum should first determine whether it is possible to get above the swelling; if it is not, the diagnosis is usually an inguinal hernia. If the swelling is arising from the scrotum, it should then be allocated to one of the above groups and its relationship to other intrascrotal structures determined. If there is any diagnostic doubt, scrotal ultrasound should be performed.

Cystic swellings

The hallmark of a cystic swelling is transillumination, but thick scrotal skin, thick-walled swellings and unfavourable lighting conditions may render this impossible. Discomfort, pain and cosmetic embarrassment are the main symptoms of cystic swellings.

Hydrocele

This is a collection of fluid within the tunica vaginalis. The classification of hydroceles is shown in Fig. 1. Primary hydroceles in adults are usually idiopathic, but secondary hydroceles may be caused by infection, torsion, testicular tumour or scrotal trauma. The fluid is usually a transudate (clear and straw-coloured), although traumatic hydroceles may contain blood (*haematocele*), and infection may result in purulent fluid (*pyocele*). Because the hydrocele fluid surrounds the testis, it may be difficult to palpate the testis, and ultrasound may be needed to determine whether it is normal.

A congenital hydrocele requires ligation of the patent processus vaginalis in the inguinal canal. In adults, treatment is indicated only if symptoms are troublesome. Simple aspiration of the hydrocele fluid is rarely indicated, except in those not deemed fit for surgery. Definitive treatment is by scrotal exploration and plication, eversion or excision of the hydrocele sac. Management of a secondary hydrocele also involves treating the underlying condition.

Epididymal cyst and spermatocele

Epididymal cysts develop from cystic degeneration of the vasa efferentia and, as a result, are always adjacent to the head of the epididymis above the testis; they are often multilocular, are easily separated from the testis and contain clear, colourless fluid. Spermatoceles arise from epididymal tubules, may lie anywhere in the epididymis, are often thick walled and contain seminal plasma.

Asymptomatic epididymal cysts and spermatoceles require no treatment. If symptoms are troublesome, surgical removal of all the cysts should be performed, but there is a potential to produce infertility with bilateral procedures. Aspiration may be performed in those patients not deemed fit for surgery.

Solid swellings

A solid mass in the body of the testis should be regarded as a testicular tumour until proved otherwise by ultrasound and/or

Table 1 **Classification of scrotal swellings**			
Cystic	**Solid**	**Inflammatory**	**Miscellaneous**
Hydrocele	Tumour	Epididymitis	Idiopathic scrotal oedema
Epididymal cyst	Tuberculosis	Orchitis	Sperm granuloma
Spermatocele	Syphilis	Torsion of the testis	Varicocele
		Torsion of a testicular appendage	Calcific 'pearls'
			Fibrous tunical nodules

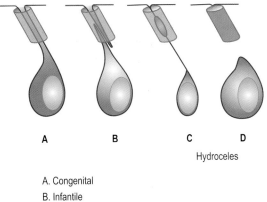

Hydroceles

A. Congenital
B. Infantile
C. Encysted hydrocele of the cord
D. The vaginal hydrocele (primary and secondary)

Fig. 1 **Classification of hydroceles.**

orchidectomy; 90% of solid tumours in the body of the testis are malignant. The management of testicular cancer is discussed on pp. 132 and 133. Other solid swellings include tuberculous epididymo-orchitis (see pp. 34 and 35) and syphilitic gumma of the testis.

Syphilitic gumma is rare and presents as a painless mass replacing the testis. It is usually associated with other manifestations of secondary or tertiary syphilis. Management is with appropriate antisyphilitic treatment (see pp. 38 and 39) and orchidectomy if needed.

Inflammatory swellings

Epididymitis and *orchitis* are discussed on pp. 32 and 33.

Torsion of the testis

Acute testicular pain should be regarded as torsion of the testis until proved otherwise and is a urological emergency. Torsion can occur at any age but is commonest between 10 and 16 years. It is caused by abnormally high investment of the tunica vaginalis allowing the testis to rotate (Fig. 2), and this predisposition is invariably bilateral; for similar reasons, undescended testes are more prone to torsion. Neonatal torsion is rare but occurs outside the tunica vaginalis.

Torsion results in oedema of the spermatic cord, obstruction of venous return and eventual arterial infarction of the testis. It presents with testicular or abdominal pain, nausea and, often, with a history of previous short-lived

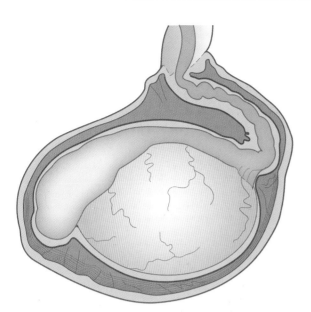

Fig. 2 **Bell-clapper (horizontal) testis.**

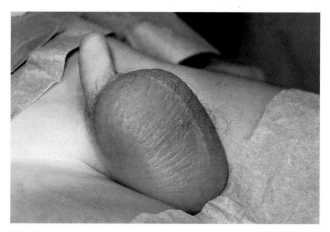

Fig. 4 **Idiopathic scrotal oedema.**

attacks. The scrotum is usually swollen and inflamed with a high-lying, tender testis. Scrotal exploration is the most reliable diagnostic test and should be performed urgently; any delay beyond 4 h after the onset of symptoms increases the likelihood of testicular infarction.

At surgery, the spermatic cord should be untwisted and the viability of the testis assessed. An infarcted testis requires removal, but a viable testis should be fixed with at least two sutures to the scrotal wall while the tunical sac is eliminated by plication. The contralateral testis should also be explored and fixed in the same way; this is not needed in neonatal torsion.

Torsion of a testicular/epididymal appendage

This affects a pedunculated appendix testis (hydatid of Morgagni; the cranial remnant of the paramesonephric duct) or, less commonly, the appendix epididymis (the cranial remnant of the mesonephric duct). Symptoms are indistinguishable from torsion of the testis, but an infarcted appendage may be visible as a blue dot through the scrotal skin

(Fig. 3). Scrotal exploration is usually needed, and the hydatid should be excised; testicular fixation and contralateral exploration are unnecessary. Conservative management is possible if the diagnosis is clear; an infarcted appendix testis eventually falls off with relief of pain and the formation of a 'calcified pearl' in the tunical sac.

Miscellaneous swellings

Idiopathic scrotal oedema is a rare condition, probably of infective origin, causing oedema of the scrotal skin, groins and thigh (Fig. 4); the scrotal contents are palpably normal. Surgical exploration may be needed to exclude torsion, but the condition is self-limiting.

Varicocele is discussed on pp. 16, 17, 112 and 113.

Sperm granulomas are usually seen after vasectomy and are found in the vas deferens itself or in the body of the epididymis. They may cause significant pain which merits local, surgical excision.

Fibrous tunical nodules

These are found on the surface of the testis, arising from the tunica albuginea. No treatment is needed, but ultrasound is advisable to exclude a testicular tumour

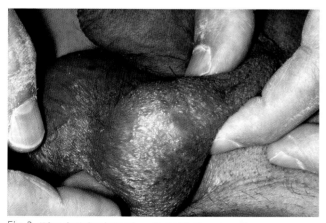

Fig. 3 **'Blue dot' sign in torsion of a testicular appendage.**

> *Key points*
>
> - It is possible to 'get above' a true scrotal swelling; such swellings may be cystic, inflammatory or solid.
>
> - In cases of diagnostic doubt, scrotal ultrasound is the investigation of choice.
>
> - Benign cystic swellings require treatment only if they are symptomatic or if they cause cosmetic embarrassment.
>
> - Acute, unilateral testicular pain in children should be regarded as torsion of the testis until proved otherwise by scrotal exploration; in adults, torsion is less likely and epididymitis or orchitis should be considered.
>
> - Solid testicular swellings are due to testicular cancer in 90% of cases.

Erectile dysfunction

Erectile dysfunction is the inability to obtain or maintain an erection sufficient for penetration and for the satisfaction of both sexual partners. Erectile dysfunction becomes increasingly common with advancing age.

History

A full sexual and medical history is essential. It is important to determine whether an organic or psychogenic cause is more likely using specific aspects of the clinical history (Table 1). Loss of libido (sex drive) suggests either hormone deficiency or a psychogenic origin. Smoking, alcohol consumption and drug consumption (Table 2) are important in assessing erectile dysfunction. Previous operations (radical excision of pelvic malignancy, transurethral prostatectomy) carry a risk of damaging the erectile nerves. The main causes of erectile dysfunction are shown in Table 3.

Symptom questionnaires (see Appendix, pp. 147 and 148) are useful to introduce the topic with patients, and an assessment of the couple's expectations is important in determining optimum treatment.

Examination

A full clinical examination is essential with particular attention to secondary sexual characteristics, blood pressure, cardiovascular status, peripheral arterial pulses and the neurological system. The sacral (S2, S3, S4) reflexes are tested by eliciting the anal and bulbospongiosus reflexes. Rectal examination may reveal a rectal or prostatic carcinoma invading the cavernous nerves. Careful examination of the genitalia, including palpation of the penis, is essential to exclude treatable physical causes of erectile dysfunction; the presence of small testes, especially when associated with reduced libido, may suggest an underlying endocrine deficiency.

Investigations

- Mandatory
  Exclude diabetes mellitus (by urine or blood testing)
- Desirable
  Plasma gonadotrophins (follicle-stimulating hormone, luteinising hormone) and thyroid-stimulating hormone
  Testosterone and prolactin (mandatory if testes are small or libido is reduced)

- Optional
  Diagnostic intrapenile alprostadil injection
  Cavernosography/cavernosometry
  Doppler penile blood flow measurements
  Nocturnal penile tumescence studies
  Pelvic arteriography

Management

All management discussions should be conducted with the couple to obtain good cooperation with proposed treatment schedules. If a treatable physical abnormality (e.g. phimosis, painful penis, Peyronie's disease, short penile frenulum) is found, this should be rectified initially. Any hormone deficiency should be treated appropriately. General advice about stopping smoking, reducing alcohol consumption and cessation of implicated drugs may result in improvement without the need for further intervention.

Should these measures fail, oral therapy is the optimum initial treatment (Table 4). Phosphodiesterase type 5 (PDE-5) inhibitors are used in most patients and are effective in 70–80%, regardless of the underlying problem. Sexual stimulation is required to obtain erection using these drugs, and they should not be taken with alcohol or after a large, fatty meal. Side-effects (facial flushing, myalgia, indigestion, blue–green visual discoloration) are troublesome in 15% of patients.

The only major contraindication to PDE inhibitors is the consumption of nitrates (glyceryl trinitrate or isosorbide for angina) because of the risk of vasodilatation and hypotension. If treatment is contraindicated, sublingual apomorphine should be considered, but it is effective in only 30% of patients.

Physical therapy

Physical treatment is indicated if a specific underlying problem is identified, if oral therapy is ineffective and if PDE-5 inhibitors cause severe side-effects or are contraindicated.

Table 1 **Characteristics of organic and psychogenic erectile dysfunction**

Clinical feature	Organic (75%)	Psychogenic (25%)
Speed of onset	Gradual (progressive)	Sudden (isolated event)
Circumstances	All	Situation specific
Waking and nocturnal erections	Impaired	Normal
Libido and ejaculation	Normal	Normal or impaired
Relationship problems	No	Yes
Sexual development	Normal	Abnormal

Table 2 **Drugs causing erectile dysfunction**

Class	Examples
Tranquillisers	Phenothiazines
	Benzodiazepines
Antidepressants	Tricyclics
	Monoamine oxidase inhibitors
	Fluoxetine
Antihypertensives	β-Blockers
	Thiazide diuretics
Miscellaneous	Antiandrogens
	Clofibrate
	Cimetidine
	Digoxin
	Indomethacin
Recreational	Marijuana
	Cocaine
	Heroin

Penile injections

Self-administered penile injections of prostaglandin E1 (alprostadil) produce good erections, provided penile blood flow is adequate, and are well tolerated by 65–85% of patients. The main risks are penile haematoma (11%), pain during injection (8%), penile fibrosis (3%) and priapism (3%). In the event of an erection lasting more than 4 h, patients must return to hospital for urgent decompression.

Medicated urethral system for erection (MUSE)

This involves insertion of a pellet of alprostadil into the urethral orifice using a special applicator. The drug is absorbed into the corpora cavernosa over 30 min to produce erection. MUSE is effective in only 20–30% of patients.

Vacuum erection assistance devices

Vacuum devices are simple and safe, but the technique can be difficult to master. They allow erection for up to 45 min but restrict ejaculation in 40% of patients and may result in petechiae or bruising on the penis.

Penile prostheses (Fig. 1)

Penile prostheses are the best option when other forms of treatment have failed. The main problems are mechanical failure, infection and displacement.

Hormone therapy

Treatment with testosterone is indicated only if there is a biochemically proven deficiency. Less than 50% of men treated with testosterone are able to achieve an erection with hormone replacement alone, and other, physical measures may be needed.

Vascular surgery

If arterial occlusion is suspected, this should be confirmed by internal pudendal arteriography; localised, large-vessel stenosis may be amenable to angioplasty, while small-vessel disease requires surgical revascularisation. In younger men, success rates of 70% may be achieved, but success rates are lower in older men (20–30%). Penile venous leakage is rare and usually caused by coital trauma. Dynamic cavernosography shows the abnormal veins, which can be ligated surgically; the short-term success rate is 50–60%, but long-term results are poor.

Psychosexual counselling

This is the mainstay of treatment for couples with psychosexual, relationship and performance problems. Counselling alone often restores sexual function, but additional physical measures may be needed in some couples. Achieving an erection using a physical form of treatment may help some men overcome a psychogenic problem by demonstrating that erection is still possible.

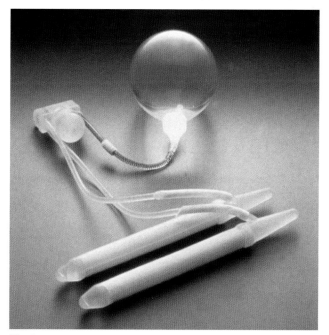

Fig. 1 **Inflatable penile prostheses.**

Table 3 **Major causes of erectile dysfunction**	
Cause	**Percentage**
Vascular disease	33
Diabetes mellitus	25
Nerve disorders	7
Pelvic surgery/injury	6
Medications	5

Table 4 **Oral therapy for erectile dysfunction**	
Class	**Example**
α-Blockers	Yohimbine
	Phentolamine
Selective serotonin reuptake inhibitors (SSRIs)	Trazodone
Phosphodiesterase (type 5) inhibitors	Sildenafil
	Tadalafil
	Vardenafil
Miscellaneous	Melatonin
	Vitamin E
	L-Arginine

Key points

- The underlying cause of erectile dysfunction can usually be determined by a careful history, physical examination and simple investigations.

- Identifiable endocrine or genital abnormalities that contribute to the problem should be treated initially.

- Further management is determined by the couple and their expectations. It is best implemented in primary care to include elimination of relationship problems, alteration in 'lifestyle' factors and instigation of oral therapy with a PDE-5 inhibitor or a dopamine agonist.

- Urological referral for physical treatment methods is indicated only when oral therapy proves ineffective, is associated with severe side-effects or is contraindicated.

- The mainstay of treatment for couples with psychogenic erectile dysfunction is psychosexual counselling.

Male factor infertility

Sperm counts are declining universally for reasons that remain uncertain. Infertility is the inability to produce a pregnancy despite 1 year of unprotected sexual intercourse. Fifteen per cent of relationships are affected and, in up to 50% of couples, a male factor is implicated.

Causes of male infertility

- Idiopathic (55%)
- Reduced sperm density/quality (30%)
- Obstruction (10%)
- Other (5%)
    - Retrograde/absent ejaculation
    - Antisperm antibodies
    - Hormonal defects
    - Genetic/chromosomal abnormalities
    - Drug induced (antidepressants, sulphonamide antibiotics, antihypertensives, antimetabolites, antiandrogens, anabolic steroids)

Clinical history

Evaluation includes an assessment of sexual performance, with particular respect to erections, ejaculation and the timing of intercourse. Childhood diseases (e.g. mumps, undescended testes, epididymitis), previous testicular trauma or surgery, chronic health problems (e.g. diabetes, chronic renal failure, cystic fibrosis, bronchiectasis), prescribed medications, recreational drugs (e.g. marijuana), alcohol, cigarette smoking and previous exposure to ionising radiation or chemotherapy have all been implicated in the production of male infertility. Men suffering any acute illness, from acute infections to recovery from a surgical procedure, can experience impaired fertility. The clearest causative factor for which men may seek restoration of fertility is previous vasectomy; 2–5% of men who undergo vasectomy request reversal at a later date.

Examination

Examination involves assessment of secondary sexual characteristics ('male habitus'), examination of the external genitalia and digital rectal examination with palpation of the prostate and seminal vesicles. The scrotal contents should be palpated; the scrotum should also be examined with the patient standing to detect the presence of a varicocele.

Varicoceles occur on the left side in 98% of affected men. They are usually visible, are often associated with a small testis and are palpable above the testis as a 'bag of worms', which transmits a cough impulse. They are found in 10–15% of the normal male population but are present in 40% of infertile men.

Investigations

Mandatory
Analysis of at least two semen specimens, obtained by masturbation and assessed within 4 h of production, is the mainstay of investigation (Table 1). A count of normal, motile sperms greater than 2 million/mL is associated with normal fertility. Measurements of follicle-stimulating hormone (FSH), luteinising hormone (LH), testosterone and prolactin are required to provide functional assessment of the pituitary hormone axis and to exclude endocrine abnormalities.

Desirable
If a varicocele is suspected clinically, the diagnosis may be confirmed by Doppler ultrasound or digital subtraction angiography (Fig. 1). Semen fructose levels are helpful if ejaculatory duct obstruction is suspected; fructose is produced only by the seminal vesicles.

Optional
Transrectal prostatic ultrasound may be performed if the seminal vesicles are palpably abnormal and ejaculatory duct obstruction is suspected. Open testicular biopsy is rarely indicated because it may result in the formation of antisperm antibodies and may cause testicular damage, which delays or precludes subsequent sperm retrieval for assisted conception. Vasography to localise any obstruction carries a risk of damaging the vasa deferentia.

Table 1 **Normal semen characteristics**

Parameter	Normal value
Volume	> 2 mL
Colour	Grey–yellow
Sperm density	> 20 million/mL
Motility	> 50% at 4 h
Abnormal forms	< 40%
Density of normal, motile sperms	> 2 million/mL

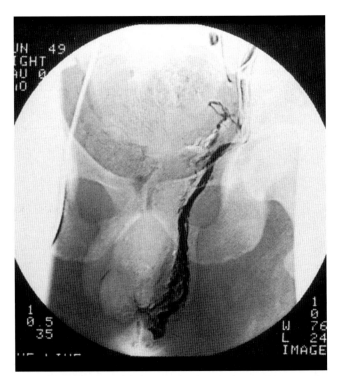

Fig. 1 **Digital subtraction angiography.**

Treatment

In all cases, treatment should be directed towards the couple and not just towards the male partner. Assisted conception techniques for male factor infertility require the female partner to undergo both investigation and manipulation.

Idiopathic male infertility

Assisted conception using intrauterine insemination (IUI), in vitro fertilisation (IVF) or, most commonly, intracytoplasmic sperm injection (ICSI) is now used. Such techniques are normally the province of reproductive medicine specialists rather than urologists. In couples treated with ICSI, pregnancy rates of 20–50% can be expected.

Reduced sperm density/quality

If a varicocele is present, sperm quality can be improved in 60% of affected men by surgical/laparoscopic ligation, transvenous embolisation or percutaneous sclerotherapy; the best results are obtained following microsurgical varicocelectomy (40–70% pregnancy rates). If this fails to produce a pregnancy, ICSI is the treatment of choice. In the absence of a varicocele, simple conservative measures (Table 2) should be instituted with assisted conception reserved for those in whom these are ineffective. There is no proven benefit from hormone treatment in men with oligospermia.

Azoospermia with normal FSH

If FSH levels are normal, it is likely that obstruction is present within the seminal tract. The treatment of choice for this is sperm aspiration, performed percutaneously or at open exploration; sperm can be retrieved from either testis or epididymis (Fig. 2). Ejaculatory duct obstruction responds to surgical relief of the obstruction by endoscopic resection of the ducts; this restores fertility in 50–75% of patients.

Azoospermia with grossly raised FSH

This is usually associated with small testes and is diagnostic of primary testicular failure. No treatment is possible, and couples should be advised to consider either adoption or artificial insemination using donated semen.

Retrograde ejaculation

Retrograde ejaculation is caused by neuropathic disorders or by previous bladder neck surgery. Sperm can be aspirated from the testis or retrieved directly from a post-ejaculation urine specimen and used for assisted conception.

Other causes

Antisperm antibodies in the male may be treated by a 6-week course of oral steroid therapy or by washing the sperm in vitro and using them for ICSI or IVF. Hormone disorders should be treated appropriately, and any implicated drugs should be withdrawn.

Reversal of vasectomy

Microsurgical reversal of vasectomy, with end-to-end anastomosis of the divided vasa, provides the best chance of restoration of fertility. Success rates are best if surgery is performed within 7 years of the original vasectomy, and the overall pregnancy rate is 50–55% (Table 3).

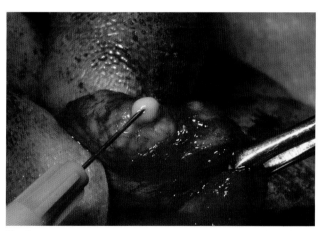

Fig. 2 **Open epididymal aspiration of sperm.**

Table 2 **Conservative management of oligospermia**
Avoid tiredness and work-related stress
Stop smoking and eliminate alcohol consumption
Treat any underlying medical problems
Stop prescribed and recreational drugs
Wear loose underclothing (e.g. boxer shorts)
Use cold scrotal douches twice daily

Table 3 **Success rates for vasectomy reversal**

Interval (years)	Positive sperm count postoperatively (%)	Pregnancy rate (%)
< 3	97	75
3–8	88	53
9–14	79	44
15–19	70	30
> 20	40	< 10

Key points

- Male factors are solely responsible for only 33% of all subfertile relationships, so assessment of the couple is recommended in all cases.

- A sperm count of more than 2 million/mL normal, motile sperms is associated with a normal fertility rate.

- Oligospermia is best managed by simple conservative measures but, if this fails to produce a pregnancy, referral for assisted conception should be considered.

- The presence of a varicocele in an oligospermic man is an indication for surgical/laparoscopic ligation or radiological embolisation.

- Azoospermia due to primary testicular failure can be managed only by adoption or donor insemination.

- If azoospermia is due to obstruction, sperm aspiration and assisted conception is the optimum treatment; when the patient has undergone vasectomy or has ejaculatory duct obstruction, surgical reversal of the obstruction gives the best results.

Appendix

NIH CHRONIC PROSTATITIS SYMPTOM INDEX (NIH-CPSI)

Pain or discomfort

1. In the last week, have you experienced any pain or discomfort in the following areas?

	Yes	No
a. Area between rectum and testicles (perineum)	☐1	☐0
b. Testicles	☐1	☐0
c. Tip of the penis (not related to urination)	☐1	☐0
d. Below your waist, in your pubic or bladder area	☐1	☐0

2. In the last week, have you experienced:

	Yes	No
a. Pain or burning during urination?	☐1	☐0
b. Pain or discomfort during or after sexual climax (ejaculation)?	☐1	☐0

3. How often have you bad pain or discomfort in any of these areas over the last week?

- ☐0 Never
- ☐1 Rarely
- ☐2 Sometimes
- ☐3 Often
- ☐4 Usually
- ☐5 Always

4. Which number best describes your AVERAGE pain or discomfort on the days that you had it over the last week?

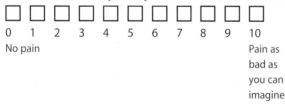

```
0   1   2   3   4   5   6   7   8   9   10
No pain                              Pain as
                                     bad as
                                     you can
                                     imagine
```

Urination

5. How often have you had a sensation of not emptying your bladder completely after you finished urinating over the last week?

- ☐0 Not at all
- ☐1 Less than 1 time in 5
- ☐2 Less than half the time
- ☐3 About half the time
- ☐4 More than half the time
- ☐5 Almost always

6. How often have you had to urinate again less than 2 hours after you finished urinating, over the last week?

- ☐0 Not at all
- ☐1 Less than 1 time in 5
- ☐2 Less than half the time
- ☐3 About half the time
- ☐4 More than half the time
- ☐5 Almost always

Impact of symptoms

7. How much have your symptoms kept you from doing the kinds of things you would usually do over the last week?

- ☐0 None
- ☐1 Only a little
- ☐2 Some
- ☐3 A lot

8. How much did you think about your symptoms over the last week?

- ☐0 None
- ☐1 Only a little
- ☐2 Some
- ☐3 A lot

Quality of life

9. If you were to spend the rest of your life with your symptoms just the way they have been during the last week, how would you feel about that?

- ☐0 Delighted
- ☐1 Pleased
- ☐2 Mostly satisfied
- ☐3 Mixed (about equally satisfied and dissatisfied)
- ☐4 Mostly dissatisfied
- ☐5 Unhappy
- ☐6 Terrible

Scoring the NIH Chronic Prostatitis Symptom Index Domain

Pain: Total of items 1a, 1b, 1c, 1d, 2a, 2b, 3 and 4 = _____

Urinary symptoms: Total of items 5 and 6   = _____

Quality of life impact: Total of items 7, 8 and 9   = _____

INTERNATIONAL INDEX OF ERECTILE FUNCTION (IIEF)

Patient Questionnaire

Hospital number (if known) ☐☐☐☐☐☐

Name ....

Date of birth ☐☐/☐☐/☐☐   Age ☐☐

Address ....
....
....

Telephone ....

These questions ask about the effects that your erection problems have had on your sex life <u>over the last 4 weeks</u>. Please try to answer the questions as honestly and as clearly as you are able. Your answers will help your doctor to choose the most effective treatment suited to your condition. In answering the questions, the following definitions apply:

− sexual activity includes intercourse, caressing, foreplay and masturbation
− sexual intercourse is defined as sexual penetration of your partner
− sexual stimulation includes situations such as foreplay, erotic pictures, etc.
− ejaculation is the ejection of semen from the penis (or the feeling of this)
− orgasm is the fulfilment or climax following sexual stimulation or intercourse

Over the past 4 weeks: *Please insert only **one** answer in box*

☐ Q1 How often were you able to get an erection during sexual activity?

0 No sexual activity
1 Almost never or never
2 A few times (less than half the time)
3 Sometimes (about half the time)
4 Most times (more than half the time)
5 Almost always or always

☐ Q2 When you had erections with sexual stimulation, how often were your erections hard enough for penetration?

0 No sexual activity
1 Almost never or never
2 A few times (less than half the time)
3 Sometimes (about half the time)
4 Most times (more than half the time)
5 Almost always or always

☐ Q3 When you attempted intercourse, <u>how often</u> were you able to penetrate (enter) your partner?

0 Did not attempt intercourse
1 Almost never or never
2 A few times (less than half the time)
3 Sometimes (about half the time)
4 Most times (more than half the time)
5 Almost always or always

☐ Q4 During sexual intercourse, <u>how often</u> were you able to maintain your erection after you had penetrated (entered) your partner?

0 Did not attempt intercourse
1 Almost never or never
2 A few times (less than half the time)
3 Sometimes (about half the time)
4 Most times (more than half the time)
5 Almost always or always

☐ Q5 During sexual intercourse, <u>how difficult</u> was it to maintain your erection to completion of intercourse?

0 Did not attempt intercourse
1 Extremely difficult
2 Very difficult
3 Difficult
4 Slightly difficult
5 Not difficult

	Over the past 4 weeks:	*Please insert only* **one** *answer in box*

Q6 — How many times have you attempted sexual intercourse?

0 No attempts
1 One or two attempts
2 Three or four attempts
3 Five or six attempts
4 Seven to ten attempts
5 Eleven or more attempts

Q7 — When you attempted sexual intercourse, how often was it satisfactory for you?

0 Did not attempt intercourse
1 Almost never or never
2 A few times (less than half the time)
3 Sometimes (about half the time)
4 Most times (more than half the time)
5 Almost always or always

Q8 — How much have you enjoyed sexual intercourse?

0 No intercourse
1 No enjoyment at all
2 Not very enjoyable
3 Fairly enjoyable
4 Highly enjoyable
5 Very highly enjoyable

Q9 — When you had sexual stimulation <u>or</u> intercourse, how often did you ejaculate?

0 No sexual stimulation or intercourse
1 Almost never or never
2 A few times (less than half the time)
3 Sometimes (about half the time)
4 Most times (more than half the time)
5 Almost always or always

Q10 — When you had sexual stimulation <u>or</u> intercourse, how often did you have the feeling of orgasm or climax?

1 Almost never or never
2 A few times (less than half the time)
3 Sometimes (about half the time)
4 Most times (more than half the time)
5 Almost always or always

Q11 — How often have you felt sexual desire?

1 Almost never or never
2 A few times (less than half the time)
3 Sometimes (about half the time)
4 Most times (more than half the time)
5 Almost always or always

Q12 — How would you rate your level of sexual desire?

1 Very low or none at all
2 Low
3 Moderate
4 High
5 Very high

Q13 — How satisfied have you been with your <u>overall sex life</u>?

1 Very dissatisfied
2 Moderately dissatisfied
3 Equally satisfied and dissatisfied
4 Moderately satisfied
5 Very satisfied

Q14 — How satisfied have you been with your <u>sexual relationship</u> with your partner?

1 Very dissatisfied
2 Moderately dissatisfied
3 Equally satisfied and dissatisfied
4 Moderately satisfied
5 Very satisfied

Q15 — How do you rate your <u>confidence</u> that you could get and keep an erection?

1 Very low
2 Low
3 Moderate
4 High
5 Very high

FREQUENCY–VOLUME CHART

This chart has been designed to help us diagnose and treat your urinary symptoms. It is important that you complete the chart over a 3-day period (choose any days to suit yourself).

You will need a measuring jug marked with millilitres (mL) in order to measure the urine you pass.

Each time that you pass urine, measure and record it in the square corresponding to the time. If you are unable to measure the amount at any time simply tick the appropriate box.

If you are wet at any time, please mark the box: + = small amount; ++ = moderate amount; +++ = large amount.

Overnight, please collect your urine and measure it when you wake up. Also, please indicate the number of times you had to void overnight.

Time	Day 1		Day 2		Day 3	
	Amount of urine passed	Leak	Amount of urine passed	Leak	Amount of urine passed	Leak
Example	300 ml		450 ml			
06.00						
07.00						
08.00						
09.00						
10.00						
11.00						
12.00						
13.00						
14.00						
15.00						
16.00						
17.00						
20.00						
21.00						
22.00						
23.00						
Total						

Name _____   Hospital number _____

Interstitial Cystitis (IC) Symptom and Problem Questionnaire

Identifying IC

To help your physician to determine if you have IC, please put a tick next to the most appropriate response to each of the questions shown below. Then, add up the numbers to the left of the tick marks and write the total at the bottom.

IC Symptom index

During the past month:

Q1. How often have you felt the strong need to urinate with little or no warning?
0 __ Not at all
1 __ Less than 1 time in 5
2 __ Less than half the time
3 __ About half the time
4 __ More than half the time
5 __ Almost always

Q2. Have you had to urinate less than 2 hours after you have finished urinating?
0 __ Not at all
1 __ Less than 1 time in 5
2 __ Less than half the time
3 __ About half the time
4 __ More than half the time
5 __ Almost always

Q3. How often did you, most typically, get up at night to urinate?
0 __ None
1 __ Once
2 __ Twice
3 __ Three times
4 __ Four times
5 __ Five times or more

Q4. Have you experienced pain or burning in your bladder?
0 __ Not at all
1 __ A few times
2 __ Fairly often
3 __ Usually
4 __ Almost always

ICS Problem index

During the past month, how much has each of the following been a problem for you:

Q1. Frequent urination during the day?
0 __ No problem
1 __ Very small problem
2 __ Small problem
3 __ Medium problem
4 __ Big problem

Q2. Getting up at night to urinate?
0 __ No problem
1 __ Very small problem
2 __ Small problem
3 __ Medium problem
4 __ Big problem

Q3. Need to urinate with little warning?
0 __ No problem
1 __ Very small problem
2 __ Small problem
3 __ Medium problem
4 __ Big problem

Q4. Burning pain, discomfort or pressure in your bladder?
0 __ No problem
1 __ Very small problem
2 __ Small problem
3 __ Medium problem
4 __ Big problem

Add the numerical values of the ticked entries: total score _____

Add the numerical values of the ticked entries: total score _____

International Prostate Symptom Score (I-PSS)

Patient's name: Date:	Not at all	Less than 1 time in 5	Less than half the time	About half the time	More than half the time	Almost always	**Your score**
1. Incomplete emptying Over the past month, how often have you had a sensation of not emptying your bladder completely after you finish urinating?	0	1	2	3	4	5	
2. Frequency Over the past month, how often have you had to urinate again less than 2 hours after you have finished urinating?	0	1	2	3	4	5	
3. Intermittency Over the past month, how often have you found you stopped and started again several times when you urinated?	0	1	2	3	4	5	
4. Urgency Over the past month, how often have you found it difficult to postpone urination?	0	1	2	3	4	5	
5. Weak stream Over the past month, how often have you had a weak urinary stream?	0	1	2	3	4	5	
6. Straining Over the past month, how often have you had to push or strain to begin urination?	0	1	2	3	4	5	

	None	Once	Twice	Three times	Four times	Five or more times	**Your score**
7. Nocturia Over the past month, how many times did you most typically get up to urinate from the time you went to bed until the time you got up in the morning?	0	1	2	3	4	5	
Total I-PSS							

Quality of life due to urinary symptoms	Delight-ed	Pleased	Mostly satisfied	Mixed	Mostly un-happy	Un-happy	Terrible
If you were to spend the rest of your life with your urinary condition just the way it is now, how would you feel about that?	0	1	2	3	4	5	6

The I-PSS is based on the answers to seven questions concerning urinary symptoms. Each question is assigned points from 0 to 5, indicating increasing severity of the particular symptom. The total score can therefore range from 0 to 35 (asymptomatic to very symptomatic).

Although there are presently no standard recommendations for grading patients with mild, moderate or severe symptoms, patients can be tentatively classified as follows:
0–7 = mildly symptomatic; 8–19 = moderately symptomatic; 20–35 = severely symptomatic.

The International Consensus Committee (ICC) recommends the use of only a single question to assess the patient's quality of life. The answers to this question range from 'delighted' to 'terrible' or from 0 to 6. Although this single question may or may not capture the global impact of benign prostatic hyperplasia symptoms on quality of life, it may serve as a valuable starting point for doctor–patient conversation.

Index